Canadian Pha[r] Exams

Pharmacist Evaluating Exam Practice

Volume 1

Dr. Fatima S. Marankan

Phi Publishing

Canadian Pharmacy Exams – Pharmacist Evaluating Exam Practice - Volume 1

Pharmacy is an ever-changing science. As new research and clinical experience broaden our knowledge, changes in treatment and drug therapy are needed. The author and contributors of Canadian Pharmacy Exams – Pharmacist Evaluating Exam Practice – Volume 1 have checked with resources believed to be reliable in their efforts to provide information that is complete and generally in accord with the standards accepted at the time of publication. However, in view of the possibility of human error or changes in medical sciences, neither the author nor any other party who has been involved in the preparation or publication of this work warrants that the information contained herein is in every respect accurate or complete and they disclaim all responsibility for any errors or omissions or for the results obtained from the use of the information contained in this work.

Library and Archives Canada Cataloguing in Publication

Phi Publishing
Canadian Pharmacy Exams Pharmacist Evaluating Exam Practice Volume 1/
Author, Dr. Fatima S. Marankan – 1st Canadian Edition.
Includes index:

ISBN: 978-0-9868251-0-1

About the Author

Dr. Marankan holds a postgraduate degree in pharmacy from the College of Pharmacy at the University of Illinois at Chicago, USA. Fatima has extensive experience in pharmacy instruction at both the University of Illinois at Chicago College of Pharmacy and the Faculty of Pharmaceutical Sciences at the University of British Columbia, Canada. Her academic, research and teaching achievements have been recognized by the Paul Sang Award at the University of Illinois at Chicago and the TLEF Award at the University of British Columbia.

Dr. Marankan is currently Faculty at Thompson Rivers University, Canada. Most importantly during the course of her education and career as pharmacy instructor at the Universitiy of British Columbia, Fatima has gained extensive understanding of the requirements of pharmacy licensing exams in Canada.

Acknowledgements

I would like to thank Dr. Al Salif, BScPharm, PhD and Samantha Sao, BScPharm for their reviewing efforts.

Preface

The Evaluating Exam (EE) is the first exam towards Canadian pharmacy licensure. The EE has been designed to evaluate the knowledge of International Pharmacy Graduates seeking licensure. A candidate for the EE must be prepared to demonstrate knowledge in four key areas:

- Biomedical Sciences
- Pharmaceutical Sciences
- Pharmacy Practice
- Behavioural, Social and Administrative Pharmacy Sciences

Canadian Pharmacy Exams™ - Pharmacist Evaluating Exam Practice is designed as a self-study tool to help the student seeking pharmacy licensure in Canada test his/her exam readiness, identify areas of strength and weakness. The book is divided according to the four key areas listed above and contains over **600 exam-type questions and answers** developed to meet the Evaluating Exam learning objectives. Additionally the number of practice questions in each section reflects its relevance (weight) as per the Pharmacy Examining Board of Canada (PEBC®):

- 25% Biomedical Sciences
- 35% Pharmaceutical Sciences
- 30% Pharmacy Practice
- 10% Behavioural, Social and Administrative Pharmacy Sciences

Most importantly, answers are supplemented by numerous comments and explanations to ensure further understanding and learning of new concepts. These comments are truly the keystone of Canadian Pharmacy Exams™. We trust that each Canadian Pharmacy Exams™ book is a valuable learning and self-assessment tool towards Canadian Pharmacy licensure. The following publications will be available soon:

Canadian Pharmacy Exams™ - Pharmacist Evaluating Exam Practice, Volume 2
Canadian Pharmacy Exams™ - Pharmacist Evaluating Exam Review, Parts I &II
Canadian Pharmacy Exams™ - Pharmacist Qualifying Exam Practice, Volume 1
Canadian Pharmacy Exams™ - Pharmacist Qualifying Exam Practice, Volume 2
Top Conditions and Therapeutic Choices in Canada™
Pharmacy Practice Laws and Regulations in Canada™

References

- Therapeutic Choices, 5th edition 2007
- Compendium of Pharmaceuticals and Specialties, 2011
- Drug Facts and Comparisons, 2009
- Lehninger Principles of Biochemistry, 5th edition 2008
- Tietz Fundamental of Clinical Pharmacy, 6th edition 2007
- Foye's Principles of Medicinal Chemistry, 6th edition, 2007
- Martin's Physical Pharmacy and Pharmaceutical Sciences, 5th edition 2005

Contents

BIOMEDICAL SCIENCES

Questions

1. True statements regarding the difference between Gram positive and Gram negative bacteria include:

    I. Unlike Gram negative, Gram positive bacteria are stained blue by Gram test
    II. The peptidoglycan layer found in the cell wall is thicker in Gram negative bacteria
    III. Unlike Gram negative, Gram positive bacteria have an additional outer lipopolysaccharide membrane

    A. I only
    B. III only
    C. I and II only
    D. II and III only
    E. I, II, and III

2. Which of the following microorganisms are Gram negative bacteria?

I. Clostridium botulinum
II. Haemophilus influenza
III. Escherichia coli

    A. I only
    B. III only
    C. I and II only
    D. II and III only
    E. I, II, and III

3. Which of the following statements are correct regarding glucocorticoids?

    I.   They stimulate lipolysis which is the metabolism of lipids
    II.   They stimulate glucogenesis which is the conversion of glycogen to glucose
    III.   They stimulate immune and inflammatory responses

A. I only
B. III only
C. I and II only
D. II and III only
E. I, II, and III

4. Which of the following hormones increase heart rate?

I. Adrenaline
II. Dopamine
III. Noradrenaline

   A. I only
   B. III only
   C. I and II only
   D. II and III only
   E. I, II, and III

5. Dopamine is a neurotransmitter with several biological functions including motor coordination. The biosynthesis of dopamine from tyrosine requires the action of which of the following pairs of enzymes?

   A. Tyrosine hydroxylase – DOPA carboxylase
   B. Tyrosine hydroxylase – DOPA hydroxylase
   C. Tyrosine carboxylase – DOPA decarboxylase
   D. Tyrosine hydroxylase – DOPA decarboxylase
   E. Tyrosine carboxylase – DOPA carboxylase

6. Which of the following hormones affect the release of prolactin?

I. Dopamine   — STOP LACTATION
II. Thyrotropin releasing hormone
III. Somatostatin

   Bromoscriptin
   agonist
   DOPAMINA

   A. I only
   B. III only
   C. I and II only
   D. II and III only
   E. I, II, and III

7. Quellung test uses India ink to detect:

    I. Bacteria spores
   II. Bacteria flagella
  III. Bacteria capsules

    A. I only
    B. III only
    C. I and II only
    D. II and III only
    E. I, II, and III

8. Which of the following bacteria are found on skin?

    I. Staphylococcus epidermis
   II. Propionibacterium acnes
  III. Corynebacterium

    A. I only
    B. III only
    C. I and II only
    D. II and III only
    E. I, II, and III

9. Whooping cough is caused by:

    A. Bacillus anthracis
    B. Bortedella pertussis
    C. Enterococcus faecalis
    D. Mycobacterium leprae
    E. Salmonella typhi

10. Acute enteritis is caused by:

    A. Borrelia burgdorferi — Lyme disease
    B. Clostridium difficile — Pseudomds colitis
    C. Salmonella typhi — typhoid fever
    D. Heamophilus influenzae — influence
    E. Campylobacter jejuni

11. Parainfluenza virus infection causes:

   I. Croup
  II. Pneumonia
 III. Bronchiolitis   & comon cold

    A. I only
    B. III only
    C. I and II only
    D. II and III only
    E. I, II, and III

12. Identify the mechanisms of transmission of HIV virus.

   I. Breast milk
  II. Sexual
 III. Blood

    A. I only
    B. III only
    C. I and II only
    D. II and III only
    E. I, II, and III

13. Identify the mechanisms of transmission of Hepatitis A virus.

   I. Blood
  II. Sexual
 III. Fecal-oral

    A. I only
    B. III only
    C. I and II only
    D. II and III only
    E. I, II, and III

14. Identify the second most abundant blood cells:

    A. Red blood cells
    B. White blood cells
    C. Platelets
    D. Neutrophils
    E. Basophils

15. Blood transfusion is in many cases a life-saving procedure. A patient with O blood type can receive blood from:

    I. Type A
    II. Type B
    III. Type O

        A. I only
        B. III only
        C. I and II only
        D. II and III only
        E. I, II, and III

16. Microcytic anemia is characterized by:

    I.   Iron deficiency
    II.   Folic acid deficiency
    III.   Vitamin B12 deficiency

        A. I only
        B. III only
        C. I and II only
        D. II and III only
        E. I, II, and III

17. Correct statements regarding the genetic disorder hemophilia A: VIII

    I.   The most common hemophilia
    II. Bleeding disorder characterized by decreased blood coagulation
    III. Caused by deficiency in factor IX hemophilia B

A. I only
B. III only
C. I and II only
D. II and III only
E. I, II, and III

18. Which of the following lung diseases is classified as genetic?

A. Bronchitis
B. Pneumonia
C. Lung cancer
D. Cystic fibrosis
E. Pulmonary edema

19. The carotid artery is a central control of breathing. The carotid artery is sensitive to:

I. Decreased oxygen levels
II. Increased carbon dioxide levels
III. Increased carbon monoxide levels

A. I only
B. III only
C. I and II only
D. II and III only
E. I, II, and III

20. Which of the following viral infections may lead to cancer?

I. Epstein-Barr
II. Hepatitis C
III. Human Papillomavirus

A. I only
B. III only
C. I and II only
D. II and III only
E. I, II, and III

21. Jock itch or tinea cruris is a fungal infection caused by:

    A. Epidermophyton
    B. Aspergillus
    C. Blastomyces
    D. Trichophyton
    E. Candida

22. Correct statement regarding the fungal infection "perleche":

    A. Penile candidiasis common in men with diabetes
    B. Vaginal candidiasis common in pregnant women
    C. Candidiasis inside the mouth resulting in painful creamy white patches
    D. Candidiasis affecting the corners of mouth resulting in cracks and tiny cuts TRUSH
    E. Candidiasis affecting nail beds resulting in pain, redness and swelling paronychia

23. Malaria is a parasitic infection caused mainly by Plasmodium falciparum. Which of the following body sites is primarily affected by the infection?

    A. Intestines
    B. Connective tissues
    C. Lungs
    D. Lymph nodes
    E. Red blood cells

24. Which of following gastrointestinal tract areas has the highest pH?

    A. Ileum
    B. Jejenum
    C. Colon
    D. Duodenum
    E. Stomach

25. Which bacteria is the **common** cause of urinary tract infection (UTI)?

    A. S. saprophyticus
    B. E. faecalis
    C. P. mirabilis
    D. E. coli
    E. S. aureus

P. aeruginosa

K pneumonie

14

26. True statements regarding neonatal infection caused by pseudomonas aeruginosa:

Candida
E-COLI

I. It is one of the causes of neonatal sepsis
II. It occurs during the first 90 days of birth
III. Symptoms include apnea, bradycardia, vomiting and diminished activity

    A. I only
    B. III only
    C. I and II only
    D. II and III only
    E. I, II, and III

Also
Candida & E Coly

27. Correct statements regarding Vitamin K:

I. One form of vitamin K called menaquinone is produces by bacteria in the colon
II. Vitamin K decreases bleeding in patients taking warfarin
III. Vitamin K is water soluble

    A. I only
    B. III only
    C. I and II only
    D. II and III only
    E. I, II, and III

28. Identify the normal range of red blood cells count:

A. 1.6 to 2.8 million cells per microliter
B. 4.2 to 6.1 million cells per microliter
C. 8.8 to 10.1 million cells per microliter
D. 12.5 to 14.8 million cells per microliter
E. 17.6 to 20.1 million cells per microliter

29. Which of the following vitamins is contraindicated at high doses during pregnancy due to toxicity?

    A. Vitamin C
    B. Vitamin K
    C. Vitamin E
    D. Vitamin A
    E. Vitamin D

30. Identify the correct life span of erythrocytes (red blood cells):

A. 2 to 3 days
B. 7 to 10 days
C. 20 to 40 days
D. 50 to 70 day
E. 100 to 120 days

7-10 days, platelets (handwritten)

31. True statements regarding hyperthyroidism:

I. Characterized by overactive thyroid gland which leads to overproduction of thyroid hormones, thyroxine (T4) and triiodothyronine (T3)
II. Results in stimulation of sympathetic nervous system
III. Symptoms include tachycardia, tremor, anxiety, diarrhea and weight loss

A. I only
B. III only
C. I and II only
D. II and III only
E. I, II, and III

32. Which of the following arteries are responsible for carrying blood primarily to the brain?

I. External carotid arteries *face* (handwritten)
II. Subclavian arteries
III. Internal carotid arteries *brain* (handwritten)

A. I only
B. III only
C. I and II only
D. II and III only
E. I, II, and III

33. Leukotrienes are biomolecules associated with several biological functions. Which of the following statements are correct regarding leukotrienes?

I. Leukotrienes are fatty molecules synthesized from arachidonic acid
II. Leukotrienes antagonists are used in the treatment of asthma
III. Leukotrienes are mediators of inflammatory response

A. I only
B. III only
C. I and II only
D. II and III only
E. I, II, and III

34. Identify all correct statements regarding the neurotransmitter gamma aminobutyric acid (GABA):

I. GABA inhibits brain activity and is primarily found in interneurons space
II. GABA is synthesized from the amino acid glutamate by the enzyme L-glutamic acid decarboxylase using vitamin B6 as coenzyme
III. GABA agonists induce anxiety and convulsion

A. I only
B. III only
C. I and II only
D. II and III only
E. I, II, and III

35. Alzheimer's disease is characterized by:

I. Formation of toxic beta amyloid aggregates in the brain
II. Decreased activity of cholinergic system
III. Memory loss, confusion and irritability

A. I only
B. III only
C. I and II only
D. II and III only
E. I, II, and III

36. The following bones are cranial, EXCEPT:

A. Zygomatic — facial
B. Temporal
C. Parietal
D. Occipital
E. Ethmoid
F. Sphenoid

37. Which of the following bases are found in RNA?

I. Adenine
II. Guanine
III. Thymine

    A. I only
    B. III only
    C. I and II only
    D. II and III only
    E. I, II, and III

38. Identify the components of a deoxynucleoside:

  I. Phosphate group
  II. Base
  III. Deoxyribose

    A. I only
    B. III only
    C. I and II only
    D. II and III only
    E. I, II, and III

39. Which of the following biomolecules are found in blood under normal conditions?

  I.   Thrombin
  II.   Fibrin
  III.   Fibrinogen

    A. I only
    B. III only
    C. I and II only
    D. II and III only
    E. I, II, and III

40. Correct statements regarding deep vein thrombosis or "traveler's thrombosis":

    I. It is the formation of blood clot within deep veins in the lower limbs resulting in partial or complete blockage of blood flow
    II. Symptoms include pain and swelling, tenderness and redness of the leg, pain and soreness of joints such as poplietal pain (posterior knee pain), fever and rapid heart beat
    III. Risk factors include heart failure, recent (within 6 weeks) surgery such as abdominal or pelvic surgery, moderate cardiovascular or neurological disease

    A. I only
    B. III only
    C. I and II only
    D. II and III only
    E. I, II, and III

41. A chancre is a sign of infection caused by:

    I. Chlamydia pneumoniae
    II. Pseudomonas aeruginosa
    III. Treponema palladium

    A. I only
    B. III only
    C. I and II only
    D. II and III only
    E. I, II, and III

42. All of the following statements are correct regarding the blood condition polycythemia, EXCEPT:

    A. Excessive production of red blood cells
    B. Absolute polycythemia is due to increased red blood cells mass
    C. Characterized by increased risk of blood coagulation
    D. Relative polycythemia is due to decreased plasma volume
    E. Characterized by decreased hematocrit

43. Clinical biochemistry analysis results of a patient affected by cholestatic jaundice are likely to show:

I. Increased serum lipoproteins (LDL & HDL)
II. Increase serum C- reactive protein ~ inflammation
III. Increases serum bilirubin

    A. I only
    B. III only
    C. I and II only
    D. II and III only
    E. I, II, and III

44. The flu vaccine is recommended for the following patients, EXCEPT:

A. A 35 years female working in a health care facility
B. A pregnant woman
C. A 35 years female with compromised immune system
D. A 3 months old baby
E. A 7 years old child with diabetes

45. Identify the normal range of fasting blood glucose:

A. 4 - 6 mmol/L
B. 4 - 8 mmol/L
C. 6 – 9 mmol/L
D. 6- 10 mmol/L
E. 7 – 11 mmol/L

46. Identify all intracellular ions in soft tissues:

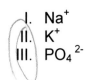

    I. Na^+
    II. K^+
    III. $PO_4{}^{2-}$

A. I only
B. III only
C. I and II only
D. II and III only
E. I, II, and III

Mg²⁺ is intracellular in soft t.

47. Who should NOT get the flu vaccine?

    I. People with allergy to eggs
    II. People who have had Guillain-Barre syndrome
    III. People with febrile illness

    A. I only
    B. III only
    C. I and II only
    D. II and III only
    E. I, II, and III

48. What is the normal range of potassium level in serum?

    A. 2.8 – 6.2 mmol/L
    B. 5.8 – 7.2 mmol/L
    C. 8.1 – 10.5 mmol/L
    D. B. 11.5 – 14.1 mmol/L
    E. 15.0 mmol/L – 17.9 mmol/L

49. Which of the following is NOT a facial bone?

    A. Lacrimal
    B. Hyoid
    C. Mandible
    D. Sphenoid *cranial*
    E. Maxilla
    F. *ZOMER* *zygomatic* *facial*

21

50. Hypercalcemia is due to excessive increase of calcium in blood. Hypercalcemia may be caused by all, EXCEPT:

A. Hyperparathyroidism
B. Paget's disease
C. Overdose of vitamin C
D. Overdose of vitamin D
E. Hyperthyroidism

51. Which of the following hormones are secreted by the anterior pituitary gland?

I. Prolactin
II. Thyroid stimulating hormone (TSH)
III. Growth hormone

    A. I only
    B. III only
    C. I and II only
    D. II and III only
    E. I, II, and III

52. Correct statements regarding active vaccination:

I. Becomes effective after 3 to 4 weeks
II. Booster shots may be require to ensure life long immunity
III. Stimulates the immune system

    A. I only
    B. III only
    C. I and II only
    D. II and III only
    E. I, II, and III

53. Which of the following is the most abundant metal in the body?

A. Cobalt
B. Copper
C. Silver
D. Iron
E. Zinc

54. Correct statements concerning cerebrospinal fluid (CSF):

    I. Turbid fluid
    II. Clear fluid
    III. Flows uninterrupted throughout the central nervous and peripheral systems

    A. I only
    B. III only
    C. I and II only
    D. II and III only
    E. I, II, and III

55. Identify the correct number of cranial nerves:

    A. 6 pairs
    B. 8 pair
    C. 10 pairs
    D. 12 pairs
    E. 14 pairs

56. Which of the following cerebral hemisphere lobes controls vision?

    A. Frontal
    B. Parietal
    C. Occipital   vision
    D. Temporal   hearing, memory

57. Acetylcholine is an important neurotransmitter with numerous biological functions. Identify the sites of action of actylcholine:

    I. Pre-ganglionic sympathetic
    II. Post-ganglionic parasympathetic
    III. Post-ganglionic sympathetic

    A. I only
    B. III only
    C. I and II only
    D. II and III only
    E. I, II, and III

58. Which of the following are biomarkers for the assessment of cardiac muscle injury?

I. Glycogen phosphorylase (GPBB)
II. Creatine kinase (CK-MB)
III. Lactate dehydrogenase (LDH)

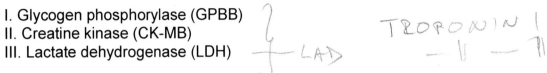

A. I only
B. III only
C. I and II only
D. II and III only
E. I, II, and III

59. Glucose aerobic metabolism result in the production of:

A. $CO_2 + H_2O$
B. $O_2 + H_2O$
C. Lactic acid
D. Glycolic acid
E. Glycogen

60. Homeostatis which is a set of biological processes designed to maintain equilibrium. Identify all correct statements regarding homeostatis:

I. The release of hormones is a key regulatory process in homeostatis
II. Most diseases are due to homeostatis imbalance
III. Homeostatis relies on three key components: receptor, stimulus and effector

A. I only
B. III only
C. I and II only
D. II and III only
E. I, II, and III

61. Which of the following vitamins contains a steroid nucleus?

A. Vitamin K
B. Vitamin C
C. Vitamin D
D. Vitamin E
E. Vitamin B3

62. Which of the following vitamins is a structural component of coenzyme A (CoA)?

A. Panthothenic acid
B. Ergocalciferol
C. Ascorbic acid
D. Niacin
E. Cobalamin

63. True statements regarding Meniere's disease:

I. Is a disorder of the inner ear that can affect hearing and balance
II. Is characterized by episodes of dizziness, tinnitus and progressive hearing loss
III. Is caused by lymphatic channel dilation due to excessive fluid in inner ear

    A. I only
    B. III only
    C. I and II only
    D. II and III only
    E. I, II, and III

64. All of the following statements are true regarding toxoids, EXCEPT:

I. Act as antigens
II. Are degraded toxins
III. Used in passive immunization

    A. I only
    B. III only
    C. I and II only
    D. II and III only
    E. I, II, and III

65. Which of the following is NOT a risk factor for hyperuricemia?

    A. Acidosis
    B. Excessive alcohol intake
    C. Kidney failure
    D. Hyperthyroidism
    E. Diabetes

— HYPOTHREODISAM
— OBESITY , PURINE (MEAT) RICH FOOD

66. Correct statements regarding ascites:

    I. Accumulation of fluid in the peritoneal cavity
    II. Treatment options include diuretics
    III. May be caused by liver cirrhosis

    A. I only
    B. III only
    C. I and II only
    D. II and III only
    E. I, II, and III

67. Which of the following muscarinic receptors stimulation leads to decreased heart rate due to the reduction of conduction velocity of SA and AV nodes?

    A. M1
    B. M2
    C. M3
    D. M4
    E. M5

68. All of the following are biological effects resulting from the stimulation of the sympathetic system, EXCEPT:

    A. Myosis
    B. Increased heart rate
    C. Decreased GI mobility
    D. Decreased salivary glands secretion
    E. Relaxation of bronchi

MIDRIAZIA

69. Serotonin is a catecholamine neurotransmitter. The following are biological effects of serotonin, EXCEPT:

    A. Bronchoconstriction
    B. Decreases appetite
    C. Decreases vomiting
    D. Promotes healing
    E. Chronotropic effect on heart

70. All of the following are biological functions of dopamine, EXCEPT:

    A. Motor function
    B. Pleasure
    C. Motivation
    D. Sleep
    E. Compulsion

71. The enzyme monoamineoxidase type A (MAO-A) is selective towards:

    I. Serotonin
    II. Norepinephrine
    III. Tyramine

MAO B - DOPAMINE

    A. I only
    B. III only
    C. I and II only
    D. II and III only
    E. I, II, and III

72. Which of the following receptors is the primary binding site of the endogenous opioids, enkephalins?

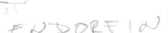
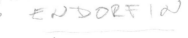

DINORFIN

    A. Mu   → ENDORFINI
    B. Kappa
    C. Delta   — resp. depresija
    D. Sigma
    E. Gamma

73. GABA$_A$ receptor is a gated ------------ channel:

A. Calcium
B. Chloride
C. Magnesium
D. Potassium
E. Sodium

74. Which of the following conditions are associated with postherpetic neuralgia?

A. Impetigo
B. Eczema
C. Pressure sores
D. Shingles

75. Which of the following epidermis layers is the rate limiting step in transdermal drug absorption?

A. Stratum corneum
B. Stratum lucidum
C. Stratum granulosum
D. Stratum spinosum
E. Stratum germinativum

76. Insect bites are characterized by:

I.   Blisters
II. Papules
III. Vesicles

A. I only
B. III only
C. I and II only
D. II and III only
E. I, II, and III

77. Glutathione is a tripeptide with antioxidant properties. Correct statement regarding glutathione?

A. Tripeptide with the sequence glu-gly-cys
B. Tripeptide with the sequence glu-cys-gly
C. Tripeptide with the sequence cys-gly-glu
D. Tripeptide with the sequence cys-glu-gly
E. Tripeptide with the sequence gly-glu-cys

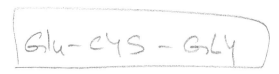

Glu-cys-gly

78. Antioxidants scavenge free radicals thus preventing cell damage. Which of the following vitamins have antioxidant property?

   I. Vitamin C
  II. Vitamin D
 III. Vitamin K

   A. I only
   B. III only
   C. I and II only
   D. II and III only
   E. I, II, and III

79. Lactose intolerance is characterized by deficiency in which of the following enzymes?

   A. Amylase
   B. Pepsin
   C. Ligase
   D. Lactase
   E. Lipase

80. Hypertrophy is characterized by:

   I. Decrease in the volume of an organ or tissue due to the loss of mass
  II. Increase in the volume of an organ or tissue in which the cells remain approximately the same size but increase in number
 III. Increase in the volume of an organ or tissue due to the enlargement of its cells

A. I only
B. III only
C. I and II only
D. II and III only
E. I, II, and III

81. Pyrimidine bases include:

I. Adenine
II. Thymine
III. Uracil

    A. I only
    B. III only
    C. I and II only
    D. II and III only
    E. I, II, and III

82. All of the following are epithelial secretions, EXCEPT:

A. Sweat secretion
B. Milk secretion (lactation)
C. Gastric acid secretion
D. Insulin secretion HORMONAL
E. Tear secretion

83. Community-acquired pneumonia is caused by:

I. Haemophilus influenza
II. Streptococcus pneumonia
III. Staphylococcus aureus

    A. I only
    B. III only
    C. I and II only
    D. II and III only
    E. I, II, and III

84. The following microorganisms cause food poisoning, EXCEPT:

A. Salmonella
B. Shigella
C. Campylobacter jejuni
D. Staphylococcus aureus
E. Chlamydia trachomatis

85. Microcytic anemia is characterized by:

I. Iron deficiency
II. Decreased red blood cells volume
III. Increased red blood cells volume

    A. I only
    B. III only
    C. I and II only
    D. II and III only
    E. I, II, and III

86. Correct statements regarding a protein three-dimensional (3-D) structure:

    I. Is directly related to protein function
    II. Is also called secondary structure
    III. Is not influenced by the primary structure

    A. I only
    B. III only
    C. I and II only
    D. II and III only
    E. I, II, and III

87. Identify the precursor of vitamin A.

A. Beta carotene
B. Retinol
C. Retinal
D. Retinoic acid
E. Retinoids

88. What is the frequency of influenza vaccine administration?

A. Twice a year
B. Every two years
C. Every 5 years
D. Every year
E. Every 6 months

89. Types of RNA found in cells include:

    I. mRNA
    II. tRNA
    III. rRNA

    A. I only
    B. III only
    C. I and II only
    D. II and III only
    E. I, II, and III

90. Correct statement regarding translation: *(in ribosomes)*

    A. Process of protein synthesis
    B. Process of DNA biosynthesis
    C. Process of RNA biosynthesis *(transcription)*
    D. Takes place in the nucleus
    E. Takes place in the mitochondria

91. Which of the following enzymes has the ability to synthesize DNA from RNA?

    A. RNA polymerase
    B. Reverse transcriptase
    C. DNA lyase
    D. DNA ligase
    E. DNA polymerase

92. Correct statements regarding the amino acid tryptophan:

I. Largest amino acid
II. Contains an indole ring
III. Precursor of serotonin

    A. I only
    B. III only
    C. I and II only
    D. II and III only
    E. I, II, and III

93. Correct statement regarding the body movement adduction:

    A. Movement that decreases the angle between two body parts (Flexion)
    B. Movement that increases the angle between two body parts (extension)
    C. Circular movement of body part
    D. Movement of body parts towards the mid line
    E. Movement of the body parts away from the mid line

94. Correct statement regarding midsagittal body plane:

    A. Separates the body into unequal right and left parts (parasagittal)
    B. Separates the body into anterior and posterior parts (coronal)
    C. Separates the body into equal right and left parts
    D. Separates the body into upper and lower parts (transverse)

95. All of the following are viral infections, EXCEPT:

A. Typhoid fever
B. Varicella
C. Cold sores
D. Measles
E. Mumps

96. Which of the following is the most abundant antibody in blood?

    A. IgM
    B. IgE
    C. IgG
    D. IgA

97. IgE is an antibody that acts as mediator of allergic reactions. Such reactions as classified as:

    A. Type I hypersensitivity
    B. Type II hypersensitivity
    C. Type III hypersensitivity
    D. Type IV hypersensitivity
    E. Type V hypersensitivity

98. Which of the following conditions is an example of type I hypersensitivity?

    A. Lupus III
    B. Contact dermatitis IV
    C. Grave's disease
    D. Hemolytic anemia II   & HASHIMOTO
    E. Asthma

99. Which of the following biomolecules induces pain?

    A. Thrombin
    B. Plasmin
    C. Bradykinin
    D. Fibrin
    E. Renin

100. Correct statement regarding tricuspid valve:

    A. Found between the right atrium and the left atrium
    B. Found between the right atrium and the right ventricle
    C. Found between the left atrium and the left ventricle
    D. Found between the right ventricle and the left ventricle

34

101. An electrocardiogram (ECG) represents the electrical current moving through the heart during a heartbeat. Which of the following defines the QRS complex on the ECG?

A. Recovery wave
B. Activation of the atria
C. Activation of the ventricles
D. Electrical conduction from AV node to Bundle of His and then to Purkinje Fibers
E. Duration of ventricles depolarization

102. Which of the following areas of the nephron is the site of action of vasopressin?

A. Loop of Henle
B. Proximal convoluted tubule
C. Bowman's capsule
D. Distal convoluted tubule
E. Collecting duct

103. All of the following are functions of insulin, EXCEPT:

A. Fat-sparing effect
B. Stimulates fat metabolism
C. Stimulates fatty acids biosynthesis in the liver
D. Facilitates glucose uptake by adipose tissues, liver and muscles
E. Stimulates the liver to store glucose in the form of glycogen

104. Which of the following fasting glucose level is used for the diagnosis of diabetes?

A. > 5 mmol/L
B. > 6.5 mmol/L
C. > 7 mmol/L
D. > 8.5 mmol/L
E. > 9 mmol/L

105. Which of the following classes of eicosanoids is primarily produced in platelets?

A. Thromboxanes
B. Prostacyclins
C. Prostaglandins
D. Leukotrienes

106. Correct statements concerning cones:

I. Cone vision operates in relatively bright light
II. Cones are localized in a small area called fovea
III. Cone vision provide sharp and colorful images

A. I only
B. III only
C. I and II only
D. II and III only
E. I, II, and III

107. Eardrum is also called:

A. Middle ear
B. Inner ear
C. Auditory canal
D. Pina
E. Tympanic membrane

108. Ossicles are three small bones found in which of the following body parts?

A. Back
B. Knee
C. Ear
D. Skull
E. Face

109. All of the following are components of a nerve cell, EXCEPT:

    A. Dendrite
    B. Cell body
    C. Axon
    D. Synapse
    E. Myelin sheath

110. Which of the following hormone is secreted by the adrenal cortex gland?

    A. Aldosterone
    B. Renin
    C. Prolactin
    D. Calcitonin
    E. Epinephrine — adrenal medulla

111. Which of the following hormones are secreted by the pancreas?

    I. Insulin
    II. Glucagon
    III. Somatostatin

    A. I only
    B. III only
    C. I and II only
    D. II and III only
    E. I, II, and III

112. All of the following are steroid hormones, EXCEPT:

A. Aldosterone
B. Cortisol
C. Vasopressin
D. Progesterone
E. Calcitriol

113. Which of the following hormones is NOT secreted by the hypothalamus?

    A. Dopamine
    B. Oxytocin
    C. Growth hormone releasing hormone
    D. Vasopressin
    E. Melatonin

114. Which of the following hormones is produced by the posterior pituitary gland?

    A. Growth hormone
    B. Thyroid-stimulating hormone
    C. Prolactin
    D. Vasopressin
    E. Luteinizing hormone

115. Parathyroid hormone (PTH) is a peptide hormone produced by parathyroid gland. Which of the following statements is NOT correct regarding the biological functions of PTH?

    A. Stimulates the activation of vitamin D in kidneys
    B. Increases the level of calcium in blood by stimulating the activity of osteoblasts
    C. Enhances the reabsorption of calcium in kidneys
    D. Increases the level of phosphate in blood by stimulating the activity of osteoclasts
    E. Inhibits the reabsorption of phosphate in kidneys

116. All of the following are autoimmune disorders, EXCEPT:

A. Grave's disease
B. Lupus
C. Hashimoto's disease
D. Myasthenia gravis
E. Type II diabetes

117. Which of the following conditions is NOT classified as an autoimmune disorder?

    A. Osteoarthritis
    B. Hemolytic anemia
    C. Pernicious anemia
    D. Sjogren's syndrome
    E. Vitiligo

118. The skin consists of layers called:

I. Dermis
II. Hypodermis
III. Epidermis

    A. I only
    B. III only
    C. I and II only
    D. II and III only
    E. I, II, and III

119. Which of the following steroid hormones contains an aromatic ring?

    A. Progesterone
    B. Testosterone
    C. Estradiol
    D. Cortisol
    E. Aldosterone

120. Dopamine, norepinephrine and epinephrine are called collectively catecholamines. Which of the following amino acids is the precursor of these neurotransmitters?

    A. Arginine
    B. Tyrosine
    C. Tryptophan
    D. Glutamic acid
    E. Histidine

121. Eicosanoids are biomolecules derived from polyunsaturated fatty acids. Which of the following eicosanoids lacks a ring in its chemical structure?

    A. Prostaglandins
    B. Leukotrienes
    C. Prostacyclins
    D. Thromboxanes

122. Which of the following prostaglandins is pyrogenic (fever inducer)?

    A. PGD2
    B. PGE1
    C. PGE2
    D. PGF2
    E. PGI2

123. Diabetes insipidus is characterized by:

    A. Lack of insulin
    B. Insulin resistance
    C. Lack of antidiuretic hormone
    D. Lack of aldosterone
    E. High levels of ketone bodies

124. Low level of thyroid stimulating hormone is characteristic of:

    I. Grave's disease
    II. Hashimoto's disease
    III. Myxedema

    A. I only
    B. III only
    C. I and II only
    D. II and III only
    E. I, II, and III

125. Which of the following viruses causes shingles?

A. Varicella-zoster virus
B. Human papillomavirus
C. Mumps virus
D. Hepatitis A virus
E. Rubella virus

126. Correct statements regarding leukocytes or white blood cells:

I. They are connective tissue cells
II. They are involved in immune and allergic responses
III. Neutrophils, platelets and monocytes are collectively called leukocytes

A. I only
B. III only
C. I and II only
D. II and III only
E. I, II, and III

127. All of the following statements are true regarding tissues, EXCEPT:

A. Different types of tissues may be found in a single organ
B. Connective tissues are fillers for internal cavities
C. All tissues consist of same cell type and extracellular material
D. Bones are tissues
E. Blood is a tissue

128. Which of the followings in not a cell organelle?

A. Mitochondria
B. Lysozyme
C. Ribosomes
D. Nucleus
E. Golgi

129. Which of the following viral infections lead to chronic hepatitis, hepatic cirrhosis or hepatocellular carcinoma?

I. Hepatitis B
II. Hepatitis C
III. Hepatitis A

    A. I only
    B. III only
    C. I and II only
    D. II and III only
    E. I, II, and III

130. Identify the common route of transmission of hepatitis A virus:

    I. Sexual
    II. Saliva
    III. Fecal-oral

        A. I only
        B. III only
        C. I and II only
        D. II and III only
        E. I, II, and III

131. All of the following blood clotting factors are affected by warfarin therapy, EXCEPT:

A. Factor II
B. Factor VII
C. Factor IX
D. Factor X
E. Factor XI

132. Which of the following assays is used to monitor warfarin therapy?

A. aPTT
B. BUN
C. INR
D. PTT
E. FAST

133. Cochlea is a tube found in the inner ear filled with fluid called endolymph. The most dramatic difference between the composition of endolymph and other lymph in the body is its high concentration in:

A. Calcium
B. Sodium
C. Magnesium
D. Potassium
E. Iron

134. Which of the following areas of the eye contains light receptors, rods and cones?

A. Iris
B. Pupil
C. Retina
D. Sclera
E. Vitreous humor

135. Which of the following is an example of irregular bone?

A. Femur
B. Scapula
C. Tibia
D. Vertebrae
E. Humerus

136. Which of the following muscles is involved in the movement of the leg?

A. Pectoralis
B. Sartorius
C. Deltoid
D. Biceps
E. Trapezius

137. Which of the following muscles are involved in the movement of the shoulder?

    I. Hamstrings
    II. Deltoid
    III. Trapezius

        A. I only
        B. I and II
        C. II and III
        D. I and III
        E. All of the above

138. Which of the following is a round bone found in the knee?

        A. Scapula
        B. Patella
        C. Pelvis
        D. Fibula
        E. Ulna

139. Correct statement regarding bursa:

TENDON   A. Connects muscles to bones and has greater tensile strength than muscles
CARTILAGE B. Covers and protects the ends of bones in joints and therefore facilitates their movement
SYNOVIAL FLUID ⟶ C. Lubricates joints
        D. Fibrous band of tissue which connects bone to bone and help stabilize
LIGAMENT   joints
        E. Small sac lined by synovial membrane that contains synovial fluid

140. Which of the following situations would result in decreased O_2 affinity for hemoglobin?

    I. A drop in blood pH from 7.4 to 7.2
    II. An increase in the BPG (biphosphoglycerate) level from 5mM (normal altitudes) to 8mM (high altitudes)
    III. A decrease in the partial pressure of CO2 in the lungs from 6kPa (holding your breath) to 2kPa (normal)

A. I only
B. III only
C. I and II only
D. II and III only
E. I, II, and III

141. The enzyme glucose oxidase catalyzes the oxidation of β-D-glucose to D-glucono-δ-lactone. This enzyme is highly specific for the β-anomer. In spite of this specificity, glucose oxidase is commonly used in clinical assay for blood glucose measurement. Which of the following statements explain that?

I.   A clinical glucose assay measures only β-anomer of glucose
II. Glucose oxidase can also bind α-anomer of glucose
III. α-anomer is converted to β-anomer by mutarotation

   A. I only
   B. III only
   C. I and II only
   D. II and III only
   E. I, II, and III

142. All of the following are monosaccharides, EXCEPT:

   A. Mannose
   B. Glucose
   C. Lactose
   D. Galactose
   E. Fructose
   F) Ribose
   G) Xylose

143. Identify the correct composition of the disaccharide maltose:

   A. Glucose – Galactose LACTOSE
   B. Glucose – Mannose
   C. Glucose – Fructose sucrose
   D. Glucose – Sucrose
   E. Glucose – Glucose

45

144. Which of the following amino acids is the only non-chiral natural amino acid?

    A. Arginine
    B. Lysine
    C. Glycine smallest
    D. Aspartate
    E. Leucine

145. Which of the following amino acids are sulfur containing?

    I. Serine — OH
    II. Cysteine
    III. Methionine

    A. I only
    B. III only
    C. I and II only
    D. II and III only
    E. I, II, and III

146. Which of the following amino acids is non-polar aromatic?

    A. Lys
    B. Glu
    C. Leu
    D. Cys
    E. Trp largest

147. The catalytic activity of enzymes can be regulated by which of the following mechanisms?

    I. Expression of enzyme precursors
    II. Feedback inhibition
    III. Allosteric effect
        Covalent modification
    A. I only
    B. III only
    C. I and II only
    D. II and III only
    E. I, II, and III

148. Enzyme catalysis is characterized by:

   I. High reaction rates
   II. High specificity
   III. Regulation capacity
   IV. stereospecific

     A. I only
     B. III only
     C. I and II only
     D. II and III only
     E. I, II, and III

149. Correct statements concerning the functions of metabolism:

   I. Extraction of chemical energy from food products
   II. Biosynthesis and degradation of molecules
   III. Equilibration of extracellular and intracellular substances

     F. I only
     G. III only
     H. I and II only
     I. II and III only
     J. I, II, and III

150. Correct statements regarding the biological functions and structural features of lipids:

   I. Essential components of biological membranes
   II. Sources of energy
   III. Polymeric

     A. I only
     B. III only
     C. I and II only
     D. II and III only
     E. I, II, and III

151. Which of the following biomolecules is NOT a lipid?

    A. Cellulose
    B. Cholesterol
    C. Fatty acid
    D. Lecithin
    E. Omega 6

152. Enzyme inhibition can be:

    I.   Competitive
    II. Irreversible
    III. Allosteric

        A. I only
        B. III only
        C. I and II only
        D. II and III only
        E. I, II, and III

153. Which of the following are metabolic products of pyruvate in higher organisms?

    I.   Glycerol
    II. Ethanol
    III. Lactic acid

        A. I only
        B. III only
        C. I and II only
        D. II and III only
        E. I, II, and III

154. Which of the following microorganisms causes conjunctivitis of the newborn?

    I.   Chlamydia pneumoniae
    II. Chlamydia psittaci
    III. Chlamydia trachomatis

A. I only
B. III only
C. I and II only
D. II and III only
E. I, II, and III

155. Which of the following parasite is the leading cause of malaria?

A. Plasmodium vivax
B. Plasmodium ovale
C. Plasmodium falciparum
D. Plasmodium malariae
E. Plasmodium vibrio

Answers

1. A
The amount of peptidoglycan is higher in Gram pos itive cell wall which explains why they can retain the blue dye and become stained. The thick peptidoglycan layer found in Gram positive bacteria contains teichoic acids as well.

2. D
Clostridium, corynebacterium, enterococcus, listeria, streptococcus, staphylococcus are all Gram positive. Other gram negative bacteria include salmonella typhi, bortedella, brucella, helicobacteri, neisseria, shigella, treponema, vibrio, legionella, and pseudomonas. Mycobacterium and mycoplasma are not stained.

3. A
Glucocorticoids stimulate gluconeogenesis which is the production of glucose from non carbohydrate sources, inhibit protein synthesis and inhibit the uptake of glucose in muscles and adipose tissues (they antagonize the effect of insulin).

4. E

5. D

6. C
Dopamine inhibits the release of prolactin whereas thyrotropin releasing hormone has opposite effect. Prolactin stimulates lactation.

7. B

8. E

9. B
Bacillus anthracis causes anthrax; Enterococcus faecalis causes nosocomial infections; Mycobacterium leprae causes leprosy (Hansen's disease); Salmonella typhi causes typhoid fever.

10. E
Borrelia burgdorferi causes Lyme disease; Clostridium difficile causes pseudomenbranous colitis; Salmonella typhi causes typhoid fever; Heamophilus influenzae causes upper respiratory tract infections.

11. E
Parainfluenza virus infection causes common cold as well.

12. E

13. B

14. C
Red blood cell or erythrocytes are the most abundant blood cells. Neutrophils and basophils are white blood cells.

15. B
Type A can receive from O and A; Type B can receive from O and B; Type AB called the universal acceptor can receive from all blood types. Type O called the universal donor can give blood to all types.

16. A
Folic acid and vitamin B12 deficiencies lead to macrocytic or megaloblastic anemia. Macrocytic anemia is characterized by increased red blood cells volume whereas microcytic anemia results in decreased red blood cells volume. In case of intrinsic factor deficiency vitamin B12 must be given by parenteral administration to be effective.

17. C
Hemophilia A is due to factor VIII deficiency; factor IX deficiency causes hemophilia B.

18. D

19. A

20. E
Hepatitis B and C infections may lead to liver cancer; Human papillomavirus infection may lead to cervical cancer.

21. D

22. C
D refers to trush; E refers to candidal paronychia.

23. E

24. C
The colon has the highest pH whereas the stomach has the lowest pH.

25. D
The remaining microorganisms are all associated with UTIs. Other microorganisms known to cause UTIs include P. aeruginosa and K. pneumoniae.

26. E
Other microorganisms causing neonatal sepsis include E. Coli and Candida sp

27. C
Vitamin K is found in two main forms vitamin K1 or phylloquinone or phytonadione in green leafy vegetables and vitamin K2 or menaquinone synthesized by bacteria in the colon.

28. B

29. D
Vitamin A is fat soluble therefore it can accumulate in tissues. The fetus is particularly sensitive to vitamin A toxicity during the period of organogenesis. Organogenesis is the formation and differentiation of organs and organ systems during embryonic development. In humans, the period extends from

approximately the end of the second week through the eighth week of gestation. During this time the embryo undergoes rapid growth and differentiation and is extremely vulnerable to environmental hazards and toxic substances. Any interference with the sequential processes involved with organogenesis causes an arrest in development and/or results in one or more congenital anomalies.

30. E
7 to 10 days is the life span of platelets.

31. E
Hypothyroidism has opposite effects.

32. B
I refers to blood flow to the face whereas II refers to blood flow to the left and right arms.

33. E
Leukotrienes are potent bronchoconstrictors which explains why their antagonists are useful antiasthmatic drugs.

34. C
GABA agonists have relaxing, antianxiety and anticonvulsive effects. Examples include alcohol, barbiturates, benzodiazepines, baclofen and valproic acid.

35. E
Acetylcholinesterase inhibitors decrease the degradation of acethylcholine resulting in increased levels of acetylcholine to enhance cholinergic activity.

36. A
Sphenoid is another cranial bone; zygomatic is a facial bone.

37. C
Cytosine is another base found in DNA and RNA. Thymine is found only in DNA whereas uracil is found only in RNA.

38. D
A deoxynucleotide has three components: base, deoxyribose and phosphate group. Deoxynucleotides are building blocks of DNA not deoxynucleosides.

39. B
Fibrin is the active form of fibrinogen whereas thrombin is the active form of prothrombin. Under normal conditions inactive forms are found in blood.

40. E

41. B
A chancre is the first sign of syphilis. Syphilis is a sexually transmitted disease.

42. E
Hematocrit is the percentage of blood occupied by red blood cells therefore it increases in polycythemia. The range of normal hematocrit is 36% to 50%.

43. B
Liproteins include HDL and LDL, their levels increase in hyperlipidemia which leads to cardiovascular diseases. The level of C-reactive protein increases in response to inflammation.

44. D
Vaccination is not recommended for infants younger than 6 months. Children on chronic aspirin therapy at risk for Reye's syndrome should also get the flu vaccine.

45. A

46. D
Na^+ is extracellular; Mg^{2+} is also intracellular in soft tissues.

47. E
Guillain-Barre syndrome is an autoimmune disorder affecting the peripheral nervous system, usually muscles, and is triggered by acute infections.

48. A

49. D
Sphenoid is a cranial bone. Zomer is another facial bone

50. C
Paget's disease is a chronic bone disease resulting in soft deformed bones. Paget's disease is caused by excessive stimulation of both osteoblasts (bone forming cells) and osteoclasts (bone resorbing cells).

51. E

52. E
In contrast, passive vaccination is effective immediately however it provides short term protection; in passive vaccination pre-made antibodies are administered to the patient.

53. D
Iron is a key component of the heme group which is the binding site of oxygen and carbon monoxide on hemoglobin.

54. A
The CSF flows throughout the central nervous system not the peripheral system.

55. D
Nerve I is olfactory nerve; nerve II is optic nerve; nerve III is oculomotor nerve.

56. C
Frontal lobe controls personality, self control and speech; parietal lobe controls conscious sensations; temporal lobe controls hearing and memory.

57. E
Acetylcholine is the neurotransmitter in pre-ganglionic autonomic.

58. E
However, troponin I and troponin T are the biomarkers of choice; troponin I is more sensitive and more specific than troponin T.

59. A
Under anaerobic conditions the reaction produces lactic acid.

60. E

61. C
In vivo production of vitamin D3 (cholecalciferol) in skin is catalyzed by sunlight.

62. A
Ascorbic acid is vitamin C used to treat scurvy and also helps maintain iron in the ferrous state to facilitate its absorption; Egocalciferol is vitamin D2; Niacin is vitamin B3; Cobalamin is vitamin B12.

63. E

64. C
Toxoids are used as antigens in active immunization. Toxins are not used in immunization.

65. D
Hyperuricemia is an excess of uric acid in blood resulting in the development of gout. Other risks factors for hyperuricemia include hypothyroidism, obesity, purine-rich diet including meat and organ meat, and hypertension.

66. E
Peritoneal cavity means abdominal cavity.

67. B

68. A
Stimulation of the sympathetic system leads to mydriasis not myosis.

69. C
Serotonin has emetic effect due to the activation of 5HT3 receptor in the chemoreceptor trigger zone.

70. D
Sleep, memory processing, mood and cognition are other functions of serotonin.

71. E
MAO-B is selective towards dopamine.

72. C
Other endogenous opioids are endorphins, endomorphins and dynorphins. Endorphins bind primarily to mu receptors; endomorphins bind primarily to mu receptors; dynorphins bind primarily to kappa receptors.

73. B

74. D
Postherpetic neuralgia is a type of neuropathic pain caused by nerve damage.

75. A

76. E
All four skin eruptions are possible following insect bites. Blisters and vesicles contain pus.

77. B
Glutathione conjugation is a phase II reaction in drug metabolism.

78. A
Vitamin E (alpha tocopherol) and vitamin A are also antioxidants

79. D
Lactose is a disaccharide containing galactose and glucose. Lactose is the sugar found in milk, its metabolism requires the enzyme lactase.

80. B
II refers to hyperplasia and I refers to atrophy.

81. D
Adenine and guanine are purines. Cytosine is also a pyrimidine base.

82. D
Insulin secretion is classified as hormonal secretion.

83. E

84. E
Chlamydia trachomatis causes sexually transmitted disease.

85. C
Macrocytic anemia results in increased red blood cells volume or MCV (mean corpuscular volume).

86. A
The primary structure of a protein determines its three-dimensional structure and consequently its biological function.

87. A
Vitamin A exists as alcohol (retinol) or aldehyde (retinal). Retinol is converted to retinal which is essential for vision whereas retinoic acid is essential for skin health and bone growth.

88. D

89. E
mRNA = messenger RNA; tRNA = transfer RNA; rRNA = ribosomal RNA

90. A
Translation occurs on ribosomes. DNA biosynthesis is called replication; RNA biosynthesis is called transcription.

91. B
Reverse transcriptase is an enzyme found in HIV virus and is a key target of HIV drugs.

92. E
Melatonin is produced from serotonin; therefore tryptophan is also the precursor of melatonin.

93. D
A refers to flexion; B refers to extension; C refers to circumduction which is a combination of flexion, extension, abduction and adduction; E refers to abduction;

94. C
A refers to parasagittal plan; B refers to coronal plane; D refers to transverse plan.

95. A
Typhoid fever is a bacterial infection caused by Salmonella typhi

96. C
IgM is secreted first as first response then IgG takes over. IgG is also called gamma globulin.

97. A
Type II is IgM and IgG mediated; Type III is IgG mediated; Type IV is cytotoxic cells (T-cells) mediated; Type V is IgM or IgG mediated.

98. E
Lupus is type III; Contact dermatitis, poison ivy and many forms of drug sensitivities are type IV; Hemolytic anemia and Hashimoto's disease are type II ; Grave's disease is type V. Anaphylaxis, rhinitis, allergic conjunctivitis, latex allergy, some food allergies are type I.

99. C
Bradykinin is a vasoactive protein produced by the kinin system which is able to induce vasodilation, increase vascular permeability, cause smooth muscle contraction, and induce pain. Plasmin is produced by the fibrinolysis system and is able to digest fibrin clots. Thrombin is produced by the coagulation system; thrombin cleaves the soluble plasma protein fibrinogen to produce insoluble fibrin, which aggregates to form a blood clot.

100. B
The mitral valve is found between the left atrium and the left ventricle.

101. C
T represents the recovery wave; P represents the activation of the atria; PR segment represents Electrical conduction from AV node to Bundle of His and then to Purkinje Fibers; ST segment represents the duration of ventricles depolarization.

102. E

103. B

104. C
11.1 mmol/L is the cut off value for glucose load and postprandial glucose tests.

105. A

106. E

107. E

108. C

109. D
Synapse is the junction (space) between two neurons.

110. A *kidney* *adrenal medulla*

Renin, prolactin, calcitonin and epinephrine are secreted respectively by kidneys, anterior pituitary gland, thyroid gland and adrenal medulla. Aldosterone stimulates the reabsorption of sodium in kidneys resulting in increase blood volume and blood pressure. Aldosterone enhances also the excretion of potassium. Aldosterone is a steroid mineralocorticoid.

111. E

Insulin enhances glucose metabolism and is produced by beta cells of the pancreas; Glucagon antagonizes the effect of insulin by increasing the level of blood glucose and is produced by alpha cells of the pancreas; Somatostatin inhibits the exocrine secretory action of pancreas and is produced by delta cells of the pancreas. All three are peptide hormones.

112. C

Vasopressin also known as antidiuretic hormone (ADH) is a peptide hormone released by posterior pituitary gland. Vasopressin increases the retention of water in the distal convoluted tubule and collecting duct of nephrons resulting in increased blood volume and blood pressure; it is released when the body is dehydrated and causes the kidneys to conserve water, thus reducing urine volume.

113. E

Melatonin is produced by the pineal gland.

114. D

Vasopressin and oxytocin are produced by the posterior pituitary gland. The remaining hormones listed are all produced by the anterior pituitary gland. Growth hormone stimulates the release of insulin-like growth factor 1 (IGF-1) from the liver.

115. B

The level of calcium in blood is increased due to the stimulation of osteoclasts; osteoclasts are bone resorbing cells.

116. E

However type I diabetes is an autoimmune disorder.

117. A

Hemolytic anemia may be also associated with the enzyme G6PD deficiency. However, rheumatoid arthritis is an autoimmune disorder.

118. E

119. C

120. B

Tyrosine is also the precursor of thyroid hormones, T4 and T3; T3 is more active than T4. Tryptophan is the precursor of serotonin and melatonin; Glutamic acid is the precursor of GABA; Histidine is the precursor of histamine; Arginine is the precursor of nitric oxide.

121. B

Leukotrienes are characterized by 3 conjugated double bonds. Arachidonic acid is the primary precursor of eicosanoids.

122. C

Prostaglandins have several functions including inhibition of platelets aggregation, vasodilation, enhancement of the effects of bradykinin and histamine, and inhibition of lypolysis.

123. C

124. A

Grave's disease is the most common cause of hyperthyroidism. Myxedema refers to severe hypothyroidism.

125. A

Shingles is the reactivation of varicella-zoster virus in elderly. A vaccine called Zostavax has been approved in 2009 for shingles; it is given to patients 60 years old or older.

126. C
Platelets also called thrombocytes are not white blood cells. Other white blood cells or leukocytes are: basophils, lymphocytes, eosinophils, macrophages and dendritic cells

127. C
A tissue can have different types of cells.

128. B
However a lysosome is an organelle. Lysozyme is an enzyme.

129. C

130. B
For hepatitis B mostly blood and sexual; for hepatitis C mostly blood.

131. E
Heparin therapy affects thrombin, factor IXa, factor Xa, factor XIa and factor XIIa via antithrombin (AT).

132. C
INR or International Normalized Ratio measures extrinsic coagulation pathway and has normal values in the range of 0.8 – 1.2; the target range of INR is higher, in the range of 2 – 3, for patients under warfarin therapy. Alternatively prothrombin time can be measured; the normal range is 12 – 15 seconds. BUN test or blood urea nitrogen test measures the amount of nitrogen in blood and is used for the assessment of kidney function. aPTT or Activated Partial Thrombin Time is useful in the monitoring of heparin therapy and measures intrinsic blood coagulation pathway. FAST or functional assessment staging tool is used to evaluate Alzheimer's patients.

133. D
Potassium is an important ion in hearing. Inherited deafness may be caused by mutant potassium channels.

134. C

135. D

136. B

137. C

138. B

139. E
A refers to tendon; B refers to cartilage; C refers to synovial fluid; D refers to ligament.

140. C

141. B

142. C
Ribose and xylose are other monosaccharides.

143. E
Other disaccharides include: sucrose containing glucose and fructose; lactose containing galactose and glucose.

144. C
Glycine is also the smallest amino acid.

145. D
Serine contains a hydroxyl group.

146. E
Tryptophan is also the largest amino acid

147. E
Covalent modification of enzymes such as methylation is another regulation mechanism. Allosteric regulation can result either in activation or deactivation (non competitive inhibition).

148. E
Enzyme catalysis is also stereospecific.

149. C

150. C

151. A
Cellulose is a carbohydrate.

152. E
Irreversible inhibition results in the formation of a covalent bond between the enzyme and the inhibitor therefore it is the most potent type of inhibition.

153. B

154. B

155. C

PHARMACEUTICAL SCIENCES

Questions

1. Which of the following drugs inhibits the metabolism of benzodiazepines in the liver?

A. Ranitidine
B. Cimetidine
C. Rifampin
D. Carbamazepine
E. Phenytoin

2. Antipsychotic drugs exhibit their pharmacologic effects on the following systems, EXCEPT:

A. Central nervous system
B. Autonomic nervous system
C. Cardiovascular
D. Endocrine system
E. Pulmonary

3. The pharmacologic effects of cyclic antidepressants include all of the following, EXCEPT:

A. Sedation
B. Flattened or inverted T waves on ECG
C. Urinary retention and mydriasis
D. Mood elevation
E. Raise seizure threshold

4. All of the following are indications of antipsychotics, EXCEPT:

A. Gilles de la Tourette syndrome
B. Hiccups
C. Schizophrenia
D. Parkinson's disease
E. Manic phase of manic depression

5. Which of the following drugs has antiemetic activity?

A. Tetracycline
B. Naloxone
C. Caffeine
D. Epinephrine
E. Chlorpromazine

6. Identify the pharmacologic action of monoamine oxidase inhibitors:

   A. Block the reuptake of monoamine neurotransmitter in the presynaptic cleft
   B. Interfere with the metabolism of monoamine neurotransmitters
   C. Act as antagonists of monoamine neurotransmitters receptor
   D. Decrease serotonin and norepinephrine monoamines
   E. Enhance REM sleep

7. Benzodiazepines may produce all of the following biological effects, EXCEPT:

A. Paradoxical reaction
B. Tolerance
C. Dependence and withdrawal syndrome
D. Respiratory depression in patients with obstructive lung disease
E. Enhancement of cognition

8. The appropriately matched tricyclic antidepressant and metabolite is:

A. Amitriptyline - desipramine
B. Imipramine - nortriptyline
C. Imipramine - trimipramine
D. Imipramine - desipramine
E. Fluoxetine - protriptyline

9. Cholestasis is the primary pharmacologic effect observed in hepatotoxicity associated with:

   I. Chlorpromazine
  II. Tolbutamide
 III. Acetaminophene

    A. I only
    B. III only
    C. I and II only
    D. II and III only
    E. I, II, and III

10. Which of the following neurotransmitters mediates the pharmacologic effects of benzodiazepines?

    A. Norepinephrine
    B. Epinephrine
    C. Dopamine
    D. Gamma amino butyric acid
    E. Serotonin

11. The rate-limiting step in the biosynthesis of norepinephrine involves the enzyme:

A. Tryptophan hydroxylase
B. Phenylalanine hydroxylase
C. Dopamine beta-hydroxylase
D. Tyrosine hydroxylase
E. Tryptophan decarboxylase

12. The neurotransmitters found within the central nervous system include:

   I. Dopamine
  II. Gamma-aminobutyric acid (GABA)
 III. 5-hydroxytryptamine (Serotonin)

    A. I only
    B. III only
    C. I and II only

D. II and III only
E. I, II, and III

13. A new drug has been found to increase heart rate but has no effect on eyes. It also leads to significant reduction in diastolic blood pressure and relaxation of bronchial muscle. This compound would be classified as:

A. Antimuscarinic
B. Beta agonist
C. Beta antagonist
D. Alpha antagonist
E. Muscarinic

14. All of the following statements concerning the structure-activity relationships of sympathomimetic amines are true, EXCEPT:

A. Presence of a hydroxyl group in 3 and 4 positions on the benzene ring is characteristic of catechol nucleus
B. Resistance to monamine oxidase is enhanced by alkyl substitution on alpha carbon of phenylethylamine structure
C. Presence of hydroxyl groups in 3 and 5 positions of the benzene ring increases the specificity for beta-1 receptors in the lung
D. A large alkyl substitution on the amino group of a direct acting sympathomimetic increases the specificity for beta receptors
E. Lack of hydroxyl groups on the benzene ring of indirect acting sympathomimetic amines increases oral effectiveness

15. All of the following statements concerning physostigmine and neostigmine are true, EXCEPT:

A. Physostigmine and neostigmine are classified as reversible cholinesterase inhibitors
B. Neostigmine stimulates nicotinic receptors at ganglia and neuromuscular junctions unlike physostigmine
C. Physostigmine is well absorbed orally
D. A major problem encountered with neostigmine is unpleasant central nervous system effects which result from its administration
E. Physostigmine is a tertiary amine and is able to penetrate the central nervous system

16. Which of the following statements regarding nerve action potential are correct?

    I. Inhibition by a neurotransmitter causes a decrease in membrane permeability selectively to sodium resulting in hyperpolarization

    II. Stimulation by a neurotransmitter causes an increase in membrane permeability to all types of ions resulting in transmission of signal

    III. Transmission of action potential results in transfer of an impulse along an axon or muscle fiber

    A. I only
    B. III only
    C. I and II only
    D. II and III only
    E. I, II, and III

17. Correct statements regarding anticholinergic drugs, atropine and scopolamine, include:

    I. Scopolamine does not depress the central nervous system in doses that are used clinically and therefore it is given in preference to atropine for most purposes

    II. Scopolamine has a longer duration of action than atropine

    III. Atropine is more potent than scopolamine on heart, intestine and bronchial muscle

    A. I only
    B. III only
    C. I and II only
    D. II and III only
    E. I, II, and III

18. Which of the following drugs would be most effective in reversing the central manifestations of anticholinergic toxicity?

A. Edrophonium
B. Pyridostigmine
C. Neostigmine
D. Physostigmine
E. Scopolamine

19. Hemorrhagic cystitis is commonly associated with:

    A. Dacarbazine
    B. Methotrexate
    C. Cisplatin
    D. Cyclophosphamide
    E. Doxorubicin

20. Correct statements regarding the chemotherapeutic cisplatin:

    I. A heavy metal complex containing platinum linked to 2 chloride ions and 2 ammonia molecules
    II. It produces interstrand and intrastrand cross linkages in DNA in fast dividing cells to prevent DNA, RNA and ultimately protein synthesis
    III. It has high specificity for DNA therefore cisplatin has low incidence of nausea and vomiting

    A. I only
    B. III only
    C. I and II only
    D. II and III only
    E. I, II, and III

21. The rationale for combining various chemotherapeutic agents includes:

    I. Mechanisms of action are synergistic
    II. Toxicities are different to avoid synergistic effect on target organs
    III. Mechanisms of tumor resistance are different which decreases the incidence of treatment failure

    A. I only
    B. III only
    C. I and II only
    D. II and III only
    E. I, II, and III

22. Which of the following functional groups is part of the structure of folic acid?

A. Purine
B. Pteridine
C. Pyrimidine
D. Pyridine
E. Pyridazine

23. Several factors or drugs are known to affect growth hormone secretion. Those drugs that stimulate growth hormone release include all of the following, EXCEPT:

A. Clonidine
B. L-dopa
C. Propranolol
D. Serotonin
E. Somatostatin

24. Tamoxifen is an anti-estrogen useful in the treatment of hormonally responsive breast cancer. Which of the following drugs have the same effect?

I. Letrozole
II. Anastrozole
III. Goserelin

A. I only
B. III only
C. I and II only
D. II and III only
E. I, II, and III

25. In the treatment of constipation, laxatives act by:

I. Adding bulk to stool
II. Increasing peristaltic activity
III. Emulsifying aqueous and fatty substances with stool

A. I only
B. III only
C. I and II only
D. II and III only
E. I, II, and III

26. The substance which is principally an emollient laxative is:

A. Bran
B. Methylcellulose
C. Magnesium hydroxide
D. Phenolphthalein
E. Mineral oil

27. The pharmacist must always be aware of possible drug interactions. Aluminum hydroxide antacids tend to interfere with the gastrointestinal absorption of:

A. Cephalexin
B. Penicillin G
C. Erythromycin
D. Chloramphenicol
E. Tetracycline

28. The reduction of gastric acid secretion can be achieved is by blocking the H+-Na+ATPase pump in parietal cells. Which of the following drugs follows this mechanism?

A. Misoprostol
B. Ranitidine
C. Omeprazole
D. Aluminium hydroxide
E. Sucralfate

29. Which of the following drugs is a tricyclic antidepressant?

A. Imipramine
B. Fluoxetine
C. Trazodone
D. Bupropion
E. Methylphenidate

30. A 40-year-old female is being treated for neurotic depression. After few visits her physician prescribes amitriptyline to relieve her depression. Following 4 days of treatment she calls you to complain that she is still depressed and the medication prescribed has no effect. The best course of action would be to advise her to:

A. Continue on the medication as prescribed, as the drug often takes up to 3-6 weeks to have antidepressant effect
B. Double the dosage to enhance the effectiveness of the drug
C. Continue on the same dose and prescribe a second antidepressant to use in combination
D. Switch to another more effect antidepressant
E. Take the medication with an alcoholic drink to increase its effect

31. A patient on multidrug therapy developed severe hypertension after eating some cheese. Which of the following combinations is most likely responsible for this reaction?

A. Ergotamine and amphetamine
B. Acetylcholine and reserpine
C. Tyramine and phenelzine
D. Angiotensin and propranolol
E. Dopamine and phentolamine

32. An 81-year-old female with arteriosclerotic heart disease and pulmonary emphysema was found to have significant bronchospasm. Her physician prescribed theophylline 400mg every 12 hours. All of the following pharmacologic effects may be observed, EXCEPT:

A. Cardiac arrhythmias
B. Nausea and vomiting
C. Agitation
D. Sodium and water retention
E. Tremor

33. An investigational drug is found to improve hemodynamics (hemodynamics is defined as physical factors that govern blood flow) and to prolong life in congestive heart failure patients. What is the likely mechanism of the drug?

A. ACE inhibition
B. Aldosterone receptor stimulation
C. Beta-adrenergic receptor stimulation
D. Calcium channel blockage
E. Phosphodiesterase inhibition

34. AJ is being patient treated for hypertension with a single drug. After one day of treatment his cardiac output is reduced but his peripheral vascular resistance is elevated. Three weeks later his cardiac output remains low but his peripheral vascular resistance is normal. What is the likely mechanism of the antihypertensive prescribed?

   I. ACE inhibition
  II. Alpha-1 adrenergic blockage
 III. Beta adrenergic receptor blockage

     A. I only
     B. III only
     C. I and II only
     D. II and III only
     E. I, II, and III

35. Triamterene is an antihypertensive classified as:

A. Peripherally acting adrenegic blocker
B. Potassium sparing agent
C. Centrally acting alpha agonist
D. Direct vasodilator
E. calcium channel blocker

36. Which of the following drugs are loop diuretics?

   I. Bumetanide
  II. Ethacrynic acid
 III. Indapamide

A. I only
B. III only
C. I and II only
D. II and III only
E. I, II, and III

37. Inamrinone is used in the treatment of heart failure because it:

A. Blocks the stimulating effect of the vasoconstrictor angiotensin II
B. Induces blood vessels dilation to enhance blood circulation
C. Acts as inotropic agent increasing the force of cardiac muscle contraction
D. Helps kidneys eliminate salt reducing blood volume
E. Slows heart rate and blocks excessive cardiac stimulation

38. A patient with refractory hypertension (refractory or resistant hypertension is conventionally defined as systolic or diastolic blood pressure that remains uncontrolled despite sustained therapy with at least three different classes of antihypertensive agents) begins to experience lupus-like symptoms. One of the drugs in his antihypertensive regimen is suspected. What is another adverse effect of the offending drug?

A. Bradycardia
B. Cough
C. Fluid retention
D. Hypertrichosis
E. Hypokalemia

39. A patient with heart failure is being treated with a positive inotropic agent for two months. Which of the following effects may be produced by the drug?

I. Increased velocity and force of myocardial contraction
II. Antiarrhythmic
III. Slowed AV nodal conduction

A. I only
B. III only
C. I and II only
D. II and III only
E. I, II, and III

40. The antiarrhythmic amiodarone is classified as:

A. Beta blocker
B. Alpha blocker
C. Sodium channel blocker
D. Calcium channel blocker
E. Potassium channel blocker

41. In the treatment of asthma, zileuton acts as:

A. Beta agonist
B. Anticholinergic
C. Mast cells stabilizer
D. Corticosteroids
E. Leukotriene modifier

42. A patient is being treated successfully with monotherapy for his
hypertension. His blood pressure is 128/84 and resting heart rate is 98. Which
of the following drugs has been prescribed?

A. Alpha methyldopa
B. Minoxidil
C. Prazosin
D. Propranolol
E. Verapamil

43.   A drug used in the treatment of cardiovascular disease is found to produce
a fall in plasma concentrations of angiotensin I, angiotensin II and aldosterone.
Which of the following drugs may produce this effect?

A. Captopril
B. Digoxin
C. Losartan
D. Nifedipine
E. Propranolol

44. In the treatment of rheumatoid arthritis penicillamine:

    I.   Decreases inflammation
    II. Treats symptoms
    III. Slows the progression of joint damage

    A. I only
    B. III only
    C. I and II only
    D. II and III only
    E. I, II, and III

45. In the treatment of gout probenecid:

    I.   Is used for the prevention of attacks
    II. Is used to decrease blood levels of uric acid
    III. Is used for the treatment of acute attacks

    A. I only
    B. III only
    C. I and II only
    D. II and III only
    E. I, II, and III

46. Which of the following analgesics has the lowest potency?

    A. Morphine
    B. Hydromorphone
    C. Meperidine
    D. Fentanyl
    E. Oxycodone

47. Cough is a common side effect of:

    A. Losartan
    B. Minoxidil
    C. Nadolol
    D. Captopril
    E. Furosemide

48. Which of the following drugs has a tetrazole group?

   A. Propranolol
   B. Losartan
   C. Dogoxin
   D. Salbutamol
   E. Captopril

49. Mr. Jones has a long standing diagnosis of hypertension. Today his blood pressure is 172/104. His condition is considered to be:

A. Prehypertension
B. Stage I hypertension
C. Stage II hypertension
D. Stage III hypertension
E. Signs of Target Organ Dysfunction

50. Afterload is an important contributor to cardiac contractibility. Many drugs are used to reduce or increase afterload. The best definition for afterload is:

A. The amount of resistance the heart must overcome in order to output stroke volume
B. The amount of load on the ventricular muscle before contraction
C. The amount of oxygen the myocardium needs to work effectively
D. The amount of heart rate variability
E. The amount of blood needed for minimum cardiac activity

51. Which of the following drugs are used as abortive treatments for migraines?

   I. Methysergide
  II. Ergotamine
 III. Sumatriptan

   A. I only
   B. III only
   C. I and II only
   D. II and III only
   E. I, II, and III

52. In the treatment of Parkinson's selegiline acts as:

   A. Dopamine precursor
   B. Dopamine agonist
   C. Monoamine oxidase type B (MAO-B) inhibitor
   D. Catechol O-methyltransferase (COMT) inhibitor
   E. Anticholinergic

53. Which of the following anxiety drugs is used specifically for the treatment of generalized anxiety?

   A. Clorazepate
   B. Buspirone
   C. Venlafaxine
   D. Lorazepam
   E. Phenelzine

54. Which of the following drug classes are used in the treatment of bowel inflammation?

   I.   Immunolodulators
   II. Aminosalicylates
   III. Corticosteroids

      A. I only
      B. III only
      C. I and II only
      D. II and III only
      E. I, II, and III

55. Which of the following drugs used in the treatment of diarrhea are classified as intestinal muscle relaxants?

   I.   Codeine
   II. Loperamide
   III. Paregoric

A. I only
B. III only
C. I and II only
D. II and III only
E. I, II, and III

56. Which of the following drugs is NOT recommended in lowering blood pressure in a patient with gout?

A. ACE inhibitors
B. CCBs
C. ARBs
D. Diuretics
E. Beta blockers

57. Hydrochlorothiazide is used to treat hypertension. The antihypertensive effect of the drug is due to:

A. Inhibition of the angiotension converting enzyme
B. Diuresis and vasodilatation.
C. Blockage the beta receptors.
D. Blockage of calcium channel
E. Blockage of angiotensin II receptor

58. Nitroglycerin is used for the treatment of angina. A specific concern related to long term use of this drug is:

A. Up regulation of receptors
B. Tolerance development requiring larger doses
C. Development of profound hypertension when given with sildenafil (Viagra).
D. Development of AV heart block when given with hydralazine.

59. Metformin is classifed as:

A. Meglitinide
B. Thiazolidinedione
C. Glucosidase inhibitor
D. Biguanide
E. Sulfonylurea

60. Doxorubicin is classified as:

    A. Antimitotic
    B. Alkylating agent
    C. Antimetabolite
    D. Platinum derivative
    E. Topoisomerase inhibitor

61. Which of the following antihistamines has the lowest degree of sedation?

    A. Triprolidine
    B. Loratadine
    C. Clemastine
    D. Promethazine
    E. Cetirizine

62. Which of the following antivirals is NOT used in the treatment of cytomegalovirus infection?

    I. Fomivirsen
    II. Foscarnet
    III. Rimantadine

    A. I only
    B. III only
    C. I and II only
    D. II and III only
    E. I, II, and III

63. A child has ingested an unknown substance and has evidence of respiratory depression. This symptom is usually a characteristic of poisoning due to:

A. Amphetamines
B. Atropine
C. Mushrooms
D. Kerosene
E. Opioids

64. Patients with normal platelet counts and normal bleeding time may still bleed severely as a result of aspirin ingestion prior to a dental or surgical procedure. Aspirin interference with normal platelet function may last as long as:

A. 4 hours
B. 12 hours
C. 2 days
D. 5 days
E. 7 days

65. Appropriate antidotes in the treatment of opioid overdose are:

   I. Nalorphine
   II. Methadone
   III. Naloxone

A. I only
B. III only
C. I and II only
D. II and III only
E. I, II, and III

66. Which of the following drugs possess antagonist activity at opioid receptors?

   I. Methadone
   II. Naloxone
   III. Naltrexone

A. I only
B. III only
C. I and II only
D. II and III only
E. I, II, and III

67. The pharmacologic effects of morphine on eyes include all, EXCEPT:

A. Miosis
B. Pupil dilation
C. Double vision
D. Uncontrolled eye movement
E. Red eyes

68. Chloramphenicol is associated with:

I. Pancytopenia
II. Gray-baby syndrome
III. Reversible bone marrow suppression

A. I only
B. III only
C. I and II only
D. II and III only
E. I, II, and III

69. Benzonatate is a non prescription cold medication. Benzonatate is:

A. Antipyretic
B. Antihistamine
C. Cough suppressant
D. Expectorant
E. Decongestant

70. Which of the following drugs is NOT used topically for the treatment of acne?

I. Doxycycline
II. Clindamycin
III. Benzoyl peroxide

A. I only
B. III only
C. I and II only
D. II and III only
E. I, II, and III

71. Correct statements regarding alendronate:

I. Classified as biphosphonate
II. Used to prevent and treat osteoporosis
III. May irritate the lining of esophagus

A. I only
B. III only
C. I and II only
D. II and III only
E. I, II, and III

72. Which of the following statements are true regarding tetracyclines?

   I.   Are bacteriostatic
   II. Interfere with protein biosynthesis
   III. Interfere primarily with cell wall synthesis

   A. I only
   B. III only
   C. I and II only
   D. II and III only
   E. I, II, and III

73. Which of the following statements are correct regarding patients with history of severe and immediate reaction to penicillin?

   I.   Have a definite risk of reaction to any cephalosporin
   II. May be given a cephalosporin without concern
   III. Have a low risk of having a reaction to a broad spectrum anti-pseudomonal penicillin

   A. I only
   B. III only
   C. I and II only
   D. II and III only
   E. I, II, and III

74. True statements regarding cephalosporins include:

   I.   Third generation cephalosporins are generally more active against gram-negative organisms
   II. The enzyme beta-lactamase deactivates cephalosporins
   III. They are bactericidal

A. I only
B. III only
C. I and II only
D. II and III only
E. I, II, and III

75. Imipenem is a beta-lactam antibiotic which is neither a penicillin nor a cephalosporin. Correct statements regarding imipenem include:

I. It is characterized by broad spectrum activity
II. It is classified as cephem
III. It should may be given to patients having a history of allergic reactions to penicillin

A. I only
B. III only
C. I and II only
D. II and III only
E. I, II, and III

76. Which of the following drugs are generally considered to be bactericidal?

I. Cephalosporins
II. Aminoglycosides
III. Macrolides

A. I only
B. III only
C. I and II only
D. II and III only
E. I, II, and III

77. Which of the following drugs required drug-free period to maintain efficacy?

A. Acebutolol
B. Nitroglycerin
C. Carvedilol
D. Clonidine
E. Furosemide

78. Correct statements regarding reversed-phase high-performance liquid chromatography include:

   I. Stationary phase is hydrophobic
  II. Mobile phase is polar
 III. Compounds to be separated must be volatile

     A. I only
     B. III only
     C. I and II only
     D. II and III only
     E. I, II, and III

79. A chromophore is characterized by all of the following, EXCEPT:

   I. Functional group
  II. Found in UV-Vis light absorbing molecules
 III. Contains electrons of high excitation energy

     A. I only
     B. III only
     C. I and II only
     D. II and III only
     E. I, II, and III

80. A stationary phase modified with negatively charged groups such as carboxyl or phosphate groups is used in what type of chromatographic analysis?

   I. Ion-exchange
  II. Cation-exchange
 III. Anion-exchange

     A. I only
     B. III only
     C. I and II only
     D. II and III only
     E. I, II, and III

81. The degree of drug-receptor binding at the receptor site depends on:

    I. Drug stereochemistry
   II. Drug concentration
  III. Drug functional groups

     A. I only
     B. III only
     C. I and II only
     D. II and III only
     E. I, II, and III

82. Which of the following viruses are useful as gene therapy vectors for the transfer of therapeutic DNA?

    I. HIV virus
   II. Adenovirus
  III. Cold sores virus

     A. I only
     B. III only
     C. I and II only
     D. II and III only
     E. I, II, and III

83. The correct disintegration rate of the following tablets is:

     A. Coated tablets > uncoated tablets > sublingual tablets
     B. Sublingual tablets > coated tablets > uncoated tablets
     C. Sublingual tablets > uncoated tablets > coated tablets
     D. Coated tablets > sublingual tablets > uncoated tablets
     E. Coated tablets > coated tablets > sublingual tablets

84. A drug has a half-life of less than 2 hours. Which of the following dosage formulations may not be suitable for the drug?

   I. Suspension
  II. Aerosol
 III. Sustained-release

    A. I only
    B. III only
    C. I and II only
    D. II and III only
    E. I, II, and III

85. Colligative properties dependent on the number of drug particles in solution. Colligative properties include:

   I. Vapor pressure
  II. Freezing point
 III. Boiling point

    A. I only
    B. III only
    C. I and II only
    D. II and III only
    E. I, II, and III

86. If the pK_a of an acidic drug is 7.4, what fraction of the drug would be **unionized** at pH 8.5?

    A. 10%
    B. 30%
    C. 55%
    D. 75%
    E. 90%

87. The following molecules are:

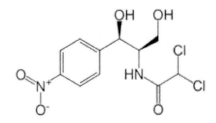

I. Enantiomers
II. Stereoisomers
III. Z/E isomers

  A. I only
  B. III only
  C. I and II only
  D. II and III only
  E. I, II, and III

88. How many chiral centres the following molecule has?

A. 2
B. 3
C. 4
D. 5
E. 6

89. The production of mercapturic acid results from which of the following phase II reactions?

A. Glutathione conjugation
B. Glucuronide conjugation
C. Sulfate conjugation
D. Amino acid conjugation
E. Methylation

90. Carbon monoxide binds to:

   I. Cytochrome P450 enzymes
  II. Hemoglobin
 III. Myoglobin

    A. I only
    B. III only
    C. I and II only
    D. II and III only
    E. I, II, and III

91. Michaelis-Menten equation will appear first order:

A. When the substrate concentration is much smaller than K_m
B. When the substrate concentration is much larger than K_m
C. When V_{max} is much smaller than the substrate concentration
D. When V_{max} is much larger than the substrate concentration
E. When K_m is large compared to V_{max}

92. Enteric coating is used for:

A. Enhancing the kinetic of drug release
B. Taste masking
C. Odor masking
D. Enhancing the appearance of drug
E. Protecting the drug from stomach acid

93. Which of the following functional groups is the most susceptible to hydrolysis?

A. Ester
B. Ether
C. Amide
D. Carbonyl
E. Amidine

94. All of the following statements are true regarding cytokines, EXCEPT:

A. Cytokines are immune factors
B. Cytokines are used to stimulate the immune system
C. Cytokine are used as therapeutic agents in rheumatoid arthritis
D. Cytokines activate genes that regulate reproduction
E. Cytokines include interferons, colony stimulating factors, interleukins and tumor necrosis factors

95. All of the following statements are true regarding biotechnology drugs, EXCEPT:

A. Biotechnology drugs are in general less toxic than small molecule drugs
B. The biological activity of protein drugs relates directly to their three dimensional structure
C. In general, biotechnology drugs reach the market faster due to ease of production
D. The biological activity of biotechnology drugs is predictable
E. Biotechnology drugs have a short shelf life compared to small molecule drugs.

96. Which of the following ionization technique is commonly used in mass spectrometry for the analysis of small molecules?

A. Negative chemical ionization
B. Positive chemical ionization
C. Electrospray ionization
D. Electron impact ionization
E. Matrix assisted laser desorption ionization

97. In mass spectrometry m/z means:

A. Mass ratio
B. Mass to charge ratio
C. Mass to z ratio
D. Mass zero
E. Mass over z

98. Bioavailability pertains to the rate and extent of drug absorption. Correct statements regarding bioavailability include:

   I. For two dosage forms of a drug to be considered equally bioavailable, the measured AUCs (Area Under the Curve) must be equal
  II. For two dosage forms of a drug to be therapeutically equivalent they must be equally bioavailable
 III. Equally bioavailable dosage forms may not necessarily be bioequivalent

    A. I only
    B. III only
    C. I and II only
    D. II and III only
    E. I, II, and III

99. Correct statements regarding the binding of drugs to plasma proteins include:

   I. Acidic drugs are most likely to be bound to albumin
  II. The degree to which a drug is protein-bound in plasma will affect its apparent volume of distribution
 III. For highly protein-bound drugs, decreasing the extent of protein-binding in plasma will enhance the rate of glomerular filtration

    A. I only
    B. III only
    C. I and II only
    D. II and III only
    E. I, II, and III

100. Which of the following statements are true regarding the elimination of a drug?

   I. Elimination always increases as clearance decreases
   II. Knowledge of a drug's elimination allows one to estimate the time necessary for steady-state to be reached after starting therapy
   III. For drugs that follow first-order elimination kinetics, increasing drug dosage will increase the elimination rate

   A. I only
   B. III only
   C. I and II only
   D. II and III only
   E. I, II, and III

101 . Drug X is given as a rapid, single i.v. infusion to a 50 kg individual. The volume of distribution (Vd) for drug X is 2 L/kg. What is the predicted initial concentration (Co) in plasma if a 500 mg dose is administered?

A. 1 ug/ml
B. 2ug/ml
C. 5ug/ml
D. 10ug/ml
E. 12ug/ml

102 . Drug Z is given by constant intravenous infusion to a patient with ventricular arrhythmias. The elimination half-life for drug Z is 3.5 hours. When do you expect to achieve 90% of the predicted steady-state level in plasma?

A. 7.5 hours
B. 11.5 hours
C. 14.5 hours
D. 17.5 hours
E. 20.5 hours

103. When a loading dose is administered, the **initial** plasma drug concentration is dependent on:

A. Elimination rate constant
B. Elimination half-life
C. Volume of distribution
D. Elimination clearance
E. Intrinsic clearance

104. Which of the following is an emulsifying agent?

   A. Sodium benzoate
   B. Lecithin
   C. Ethanol
   D. Benzalkonium chloride
   E. EDTA

105. Correct statements regarding epimers:

   I. Epimers differ by at least one sterocentre
   II. Epimers are diastereoisomers
   III. Tetracycline and epi-tetracycline are epimers

     A. I only
     B. III only
     C. I and II only
     D. II and III only
     E. I, II, and III

106. A 24 year old male soccer player is admitted in the emergency room with pain and swelling near the ankle. Upon examination a ruptured tendon with tendonitis setting in was found. His previous antibiotic therapy was suspected to have a contribution in his present condition. Which one of the following antibiotics was previously given to this patient?

A. Ceftriaxone
B. Clarithromycin
C. Ciprofloxacin
D. Amoxicillin
E .Penicillin

107. A patient with watery stools is diagnosed with amoebic dysentery. He is given a drug that causes a metallic taste. Which of the following drugs was prescribed?

A. Iodoquinol
B. Paromomycin
C. Metronidazole
D. Emetine
E. Ciprofloxacin

108. The amount of sodium, phosphate or magnesium contained in an antacid should be assessed when selecting an antacid for patients with all, EXCEPT:

A. Renal insufficiency
B. Congestive heart failure
C. Ascites
D. Peptic ulcer disease
E. Hypertension

109. Which of the following test is NOT used in the assessment inflammatory bowel disease?

A. WBC
B. C-reactive protein
C. Iron binding capacity
D. Stool culture
E. Albumin level

110. Which of the following is not found in commercial sunscreen formulations?

I. Benzyl peroxide
II. Zinc oxide
III. Avobenzone

A. I only
B. III only
C. I and II only
D. II and III only
E. I, II, and III

111. Which of the following values are useful in the assessment of the effectiveness of an investigational drug?

    I. AUC
    II. Absorption rate
    III. t-max.

      A. I only
      B. III only
      C. I and II only
      D. II and III only
      E. I, II, and III

112. Which of the following factors does not affect HPLC flow rate?

      A. Mobile phase
      B. Stationary phase
      C. Sample concentration
      D. Detector
      E. Pressure

113. Which of the following is not a suppository base?

    I. Cocoa butter
    II. Gelatinized glycerin
    III. Lactose

      A. I only
      B. III only
      C. I and II only
      D. II and III only
      E. I, II, and III

114. Which of the following is a water soluble ointment base?

    I. Lanolin
    II. Petrolatum
    III. Polyethylene glycol

A. I only
B. III only
C. I and II only
D. II and III only
E. I, II, and III

115. Which of the following is an oleaginous base?

   I. Petrolatum
  II. Cold cream
 III. Polyethylene glycol

   A. I only
   B. III only
   C. I and II only
   D. II and III only
   E. I, II, and III

116. In general, compared to the parent drug a drug metabolite is characterized by:

A. Higher therapeutic activity
B. Lower therapeutic activity
C. Higher lipid solubility
D. Higher water solubility
E. Same partition coefficient

117. Structural isomers are:

   I. Different in their bonding sequence
  II. Stereoisomers
 III. Mirror images

   A. I only
   B. III only
   C. I and II only
   D. II and III only
   E. I, II, and III

118. Based on the structure of ephedrine shown below, under which conditions this drug will have the highest water solubility?

   I. Neutral
  II. Basic
 III. Acidic

    A. I only
    B. III only
    C. I and II only
    D. II and III only
    E. I, II, and III

Ephedrine

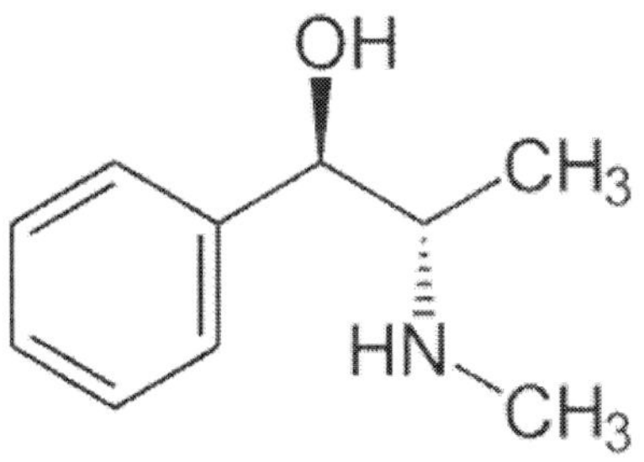

119. A drug characterized by a large volume of distribution (Vd) has:

    A. High degree of plasma protein binding
    B. High tissue affinity relative to plasma
    C. A large first-pass effect if given orally
    D. High renal clearance
    E. High absorption rate

120. Three different formulations of the same drug have the following absorption rates (ka).

Formulation	ka (hr-1)
1	0.2
2	0.3
3	0.4

Assuming that all three formulations have the same elimination rate, which one will have the fastest onset of action?

    A. 1
    B. 2
    C. 3
    D. All three will have same onset of action because they have the same elimination rate
    E. Inconclusive. The absorption rate alone doesn't provide such information

121. A patient is administered a drug as a sublingual (SL) tablet and as an oral rapid release formulation; identical doses were administered with each administration. The plasma concentration of the drug after SL administration is substantially higher than that found after oral administration and the intensity and duration of pharmacologic effect are greater following oral administration. Which of the following are correct statements regarding this observation?

I. The drug is poorly absorbed due to low lipid solubility
II. The drug undergoes extensive first-pass metabolism
III. The pharmacologic activity of the drug is related to its metabolite

    A. I only
    B. III only
    C. I and II only
    D. II and III only
    E. I, II, and III

122. What is the percentage of a dose of pentobarbital ionized at plasma pH? Pentobarbital has a pKa value of 8.0.

A. 35%
B. 50%
C. 62%
D. 80%
E. 95%

123. Which of the following drugs are acidic?

I

II

III

A. I only
B. III only
C. I and II only
D. II and III only
E. I, II, and III

124. Assign the configuration around the chiral center marked by a star.

Propranolol

A. R
B. S

125. Assign the configuration around the chiral center marked by a star.

Norepinephrine

A. R
B. S

126. Assign the configuration around the chiral center marked by a star.

Thalidomide

A. R
B. S

127. Assign the configuration around the chiral centers marked 1 and 2.

Pseudoephedrine

A. R, S
B. R, R
C. S, R
D. S, S

128. Identify the correct configuration of tripolidine:

Triprolidine

A. Z
B. E

129. Identify the correct configuration of tamoxifen:

Tamoxifen

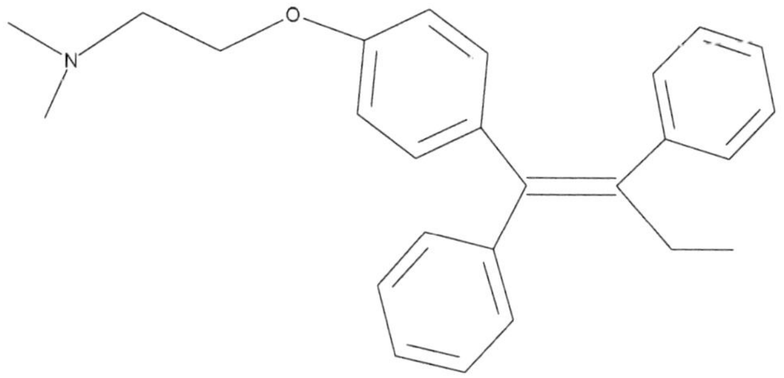

A. Z
B. E

130. Identify the correct configuration of chloramitriptyline:

Chloramitriptyline

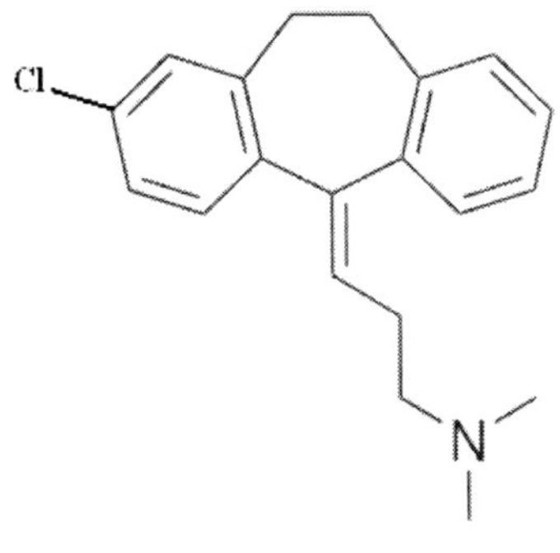

A. Z
B. E

131. The following phase I metabolic reaction is described as:

Acetanilide

A. Deamination
B. N-dealkylation
C. Aromatic hydroxylation
D. O-dealkylation
E. Methyl oxidation

132. The following phase I metabolic reaction is described as:

Imipramine

A. Deamination
B. N-dealkylation
C. Aromatic hydroxylation
D. O-dealkylation
E. Methyl oxidation

133. The following phase I metabolic reaction is described as:

Amphetamine

  A. Deamination
  B. N-dealkylation
  C. Aromatic hydroxylation
  D. O-dealkylation
  E. Methyl oxidation

134. The rate of drug absorption may be affected by all, EXCEPT:

  A. Blood flow at the site of administration
  B. Binding to plasma proteins
  C. Drug concentration
  D. Drug lipid solubility
  E. Drug partition coefficient

135. Drug metabolism may be affected by:

  I.   Patient's physiology
  II. Route of administration
  III. Drug-drug interactions

  A. I only
  B. III only
  C. I and II only
  D. II and III only
  E. I, II, and III

136. Which of the following reactions are phase II metabolic reactions?

    I. Sulfoxidation
   II. Deamination
  III. Acetylation

    A. I only
    B. III only
    C. I and II only
    D. II and III only
    E. I, II, and III

137. What is the plasma concentration of 45 mg drug dose given by IV assuming a volume of distribution of 104 L?

    A. 0.43 mg/L
    B. 0.85 mg/L
    C. 1.4 mg/L
    D. 2.0mg/L
    E. 3.5 mg/L

138. What is the half-life of a drug with an elimination rate of 54% per hour assuming first order kinetics?

    A. 0.8 hour
    B. 1.3 hours
    C. 2.2 hours
    D. 3.5 hours
    E. 5.4 hours

139. A drug with a half-life of 5 hours is administered to an 85 kg patient. The volume of distribution of the drug is 95 mL/kg. What is the total body clearance of the drug?

    A. 0.95 L/h
    B. 1.12 L/h
    C. 2.50 L/h
    D. 3.22 L/h
    E. 4.70 L/h

140. The binding of a drug to plasma proteins may result in:

   I. Increased incidence of drug-drug interactions
  II. Increased renal clearance
 III. Increased drug distribution to tissues

     A. I only
     B. III only
     C. I and II only
     D. II and III only
     E. I, II, and III

141. A drug has a half-life of 4 hours. Following administration of a 400 mg dose what will be the amount of drug remaining in the body after 12 hours?

     A. 8 mg
     B. 10 mg
     C. 25 mg
     D. 40 mg
     E. 50 mg

142. Drug dissolution may be described using which of the following equations?

     A. Noyes-Whitney
     B. Stoke's
     C. Fick's
     D. Raoult's law
     E. Poiseuille's law

143. JT a 55 years old diabetic has significant problems with gastric reflux. He also suffers from arthritis and takes enteric coated aspirin. As treatment for his gastric reflux, JT is placed on metoclopramide an agent which increases the rate of gastric emptying. Which of the following statements is correct regarding the effect of metoclopramide on the onset, duration, and intensity of the aspirin therapy?

A. Onset, intensity and duration of action will be faster
B. Onset, intensity and duration of action will be slower
C. Onset will be slower whereas intensity and duration of action will be faster
D. Onset will be faster whereas intensity and duration of action will be slower
E. Onset will be faster whereas intensity and duration of action will remain the same
F. Onset will be slower whereas intensity and duration of action will remain the same

144. Administration of an enzyme inducer that increases the metabolism of a drug that is subject to significant first-pass metabolism and is administered orally would be expected to affect all of the following compared to the drug given orally without the enzyme inducer, EXCEPT:

A. Rate of elimination
B. Rate of absorption
C. Peak concentration of active drug
D. Peak concentration of drug metabolite
E. Pharmacologic effect of the drug

145. The kinetics data for an enzymatic reaction in the presence **and** absence of inhibitors are plotted below. Identify the curve that corresponds to competitive inhibition:

A. Curve 1
B. Curve 2
C. Curve 3
D. Curve 4

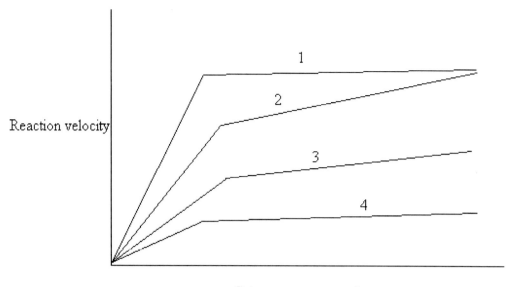

Reaction velocity

Substrate concentration

146. Phosphoglyceride A has a higher melting point (Tm) than phosphoglyceride B. All of the following statements are correct regarding the differences between A and B, EXCEPT:

    A. A has a longer fatty acid chain than B
    B. A has more unsaturated bonds in its fatty acid chain than B
    C. A has more saturated bonds in its fatty acid chain than B
    D. A has trans unsaturated bonds whereas B has cis unsaturated bonds
    E. Fatty acid chains in A interact stronger than the fatty acid chains in B

147. Identify the complementary sequence of the following DNA sequence: ATTCGTTAACCGTAA

    A. TTAGGAATTCGGATT
    B. ATTCGAATGGATTAA
    C. TAAGCAATTGGCATT
    D. TAAGCTATTGCCATT
    E. ATCCGTAATGTATTA

148. All of the following statements are true regarding tRNA, EXCEPT:

    A. It contains an anticodon which binds a codon on the mRNA
    B. It can become covalently attached to an amino acid
    C. It interacts with mRNA during replication
    D. It serves as an adaptor between the information in mRNA and an individual amino acid
    E. It is serves as mediator during protein synthesis

149. Protein synthesis occurs on the ribosomes. Which of the following biomolecules are components of ribosomes?

    A. protein and mRNA
    B. protein and rRNA
    C. protein and tRNA
    D. mRNA and rRNA
    E. rRNA and tRNA

150. Correct statements regarding the reaction shown below:

Benzoic acid

Hippuric acid

  I. Phase I reaction
  II. Phase II reaction
  III. Amino acid conjugation

    A. I only
    B. III only
    C. I and II only
    D. II and III only
    E. I, II, and III

151. Which of the following is unlikely to denature a protein?

    A. Organic solvent
    B. High temperature
    C. Salt
    D. Shaking
    E. Exposure to radiation

152. Which one of the following electrophoresis bands visualization techniques have high specificity?

    I. Coomassie staining
    II. Silver staining
    III. Immunoblotting (Western blot)

    A. I only
    B. III only
    C. I and II only
    D. II and III only
    E. I, II, and III

153. Protein separation by SDS-PAGE is based on:

    I. Protein molecular weight
    II. Protein shape
    III. Protein charge

    A. I only
    B. III only
    C. I and II only
    D. II and III only
    E. I, II, and III

154. Which of the following vitamins is produced by bacteria in the colon?

    A. Vitamin K1
    B. Vitamin D3
    C. Vitamin D2
    D. Vitamin K2
    E. Vitamin C

155. Correct statements concerning INR:

   I. Measures primarily the intrinsic pathway of coagulation
  II. Measures primarily the extrinsic pathway of coagulation
 III. Reference value is 0.8 – 1.2

     A. I only
     B. III only
     C. I and II only
     D. II and III only
     E. I, II, and III

156. Which of the following statements concerning therapeutic drug monitoring (TDM) are correct?

   I. TDM guides the design of effective and safe individualized drug regimens
  II. TDM helps maintain consistent level of drug in the bloodstream
 III. TDM is required for all therapeutic agents

     A. I only
     B. III only
     C. I and II only
     D. II and III only
     E. I, II, and III

157. Which of the following factors may result in drug pharmacokinetic variability?

   I. Drug-drug interactions
  II. Patient compliance
 III. Diet

     A. I only
     B. III only
     C. I and II only
     D. II and III only
     E. I, II, and III

158. PKU is characterized by ineffective metabolism of which of the following amino acids?

    A. Tyrosine
    B. Phenylalanine
    C. Alanine
    D. Isoleucine
    E. Proline

159. All of the following are lipids metabolism disorders, EXCEPT:

  I. Gaucher's disease
  II. Neiman Pick disease
 III. Forbe's disease

    A. I only
    B. III only
    C. I and II only
    D. II and III only
    E. I, II, and III

160. Identify the structural differences between linoleic acid and alpha linolenic acid:

  I. Number of double bonds
  II. Position of the first double bond
 III. Cis/trans configuration

    A. I only
    B. III only
    C. I and II only
    D. II and III only
    E. I, II, and III

161. Viral meningitis is characterized by:

    A. Turbid cerebrospinal fluid
    B. Clear colorless cerebrospinal fluid
    C. Decreased lymphocytes in cerebrospinal fluid
    D. Decreased glucose level in cerebrospinal fluid
    E. Decreased protein level in cerebrospinal fluid

162. All of the following are liver disease biomarkers, EXCEPT:

    A. Aspartate aminotransferase
    B. Alkaline phosphatase
    C. Glutamate dehydrogenase
    D. Creatine kinase
    E. Alanine aminotransferase

163. All of the following are breast cancer biomarkers, EXCEPT:

    A. Creatine kinase BB
    B. Esterase
    C. Aryl sulfatase B
    D. Sialytransferase
    E. Hexokinase

164. Urine glucose assay can be performed by:

    I. Clinitest
   II. Glucose oxidase test
  III. Bromophenol blue test

    A. I only
    B. III only
    C. I and II only
    D. II and III only
    E. I, II, and III

165. All of the following are water soluble vitamins, EXCEPT:

A. Retinol
B. Thiamin
C. Cobalamin
D. Ascorbic acid
E. Pyridoxin

166. Which of the following have antioxidant property, EXCEPT:

A. Vitamin K
B. Vitamin E
C. Glutathione
D. Vitamin A
E. Lipoic acid

167. Identify a non-essential amino acid :

A. Tryptophan
B. Methionine
C. Proline
D. Phenylalanine
E. Histidine

168. Identify the primary mechanism of acetaminophen detoxification:

A. Gluronidation
B. Sulfation
C. Glutathione conjugation
D. Amino acid conjugation
E. Methylation

169. Carbon monoxide toxicity results in the production of:

A. Methemoglobin
B. Carboxyhemoglobin
C. Carbaminohemoglobin
D. Cyanomethemoglobin
E. Deoxyhemoglobin

170. Which of the following values are needed in the Cockcroft and Gault formula for the estimation of creatinine clearance?

I. Serum creatine
II. Age
III. Weight

A. I only
B. III only
C. I and II only
D. II and III only
E. I, II, and III

171. Which of the following vitamin deficiencies leads to stomatitis?

A. Vitamin B2
B. Vitamin A
C. Vitamin B1
D. Vitamin E
E. Vitamin K

Case study: Questions 172 to 175

YP is a 47 years old cancer patient who has been just diagnosed with secondary Raynaud's phenomenon. He is currently under a combo therapy including cisplatin and interferon alpha. He is also using ondansetron for the management of nausea and vomiting.

172. Raynaud's phenomenon is characterized by:

A. Sensitivity to heat
B. Sensitivity to cold
C. Sensitivity to UV light
D. Sensitivity to sound
E. Sensitivity to touch

173. Which of the following drugs in the patient therapeutic regimen cause secondary Raynaud's phenomenon?

I. Cisplatin
II. Interferon alpha
III. Ondansetron

A. I only
B. III only
C. I and II only
D. II and III only
E. I, II, and III

174. Ondansetron is classified as:

A. Corticosteroid
B. Opioid
C. Serotonin antagonist
D. Benzodiazepine
E. Dopamine antagonist

175. Raynaud's phenomenon is best treated with.

    A. Nifedipine XL
    B. Vardenafil
    C. Felodipine
    D. Diltiazem
    E. Prazosin

176. Which of the following drugs is used to treat alopecia?

    A. Hydralazine
    B. Atorvastatin
    C. Sildenafil
    D. Minoxidil
    E. Bumetanide

177. In the treatment of hyperlipidemia, Niacin:

    I. Increase HDL
    II. Decrease LDL
    III. Decrease triglycerides

    A. I only
    B. III only
    C. I and II only
    D. II and III only
    E. I, II, and III

178. Osmotic diuretics act on:

    A. Loop of Henle
    B. Distal tubule
    C. Collecting duct
    D. Proximal tubule

179. All of the following are selective beta1 blockers, EXCEPT:

    A. Acebutolol
    B. Esmolol
    C. Metoprolol
    D. Nadolol
    E. Atenolol

180. Which of the following beta blockers have intrinsic sympathomimetic activity?

    I. Carvedilol
    II. Acebutolol
    III. Pindolol

        A. I only
        B. III only
        C. I and II only
        D. II and III only
        E. I, II, and III

181. Which of the following classes of adrenergic drugs are useful in the treatment of benign prostatic hyperplasia?

    I. Antimuscarinics
    II. Alpha blockers
    III. 5-alpha reductase inhibitors

        A. I only
        B. III only
        C. I and II only
        D. II and III only
        E. I, II, and III

182. Which of the following drug classes should be included in post-heart valve replacement therapeutic regimen?

    A. CCBs
    B. Nitrates
    C. ACE inhibitors
    D. Anticoagulants
    E. Alpha-blockers

183. The pharmacologic effects produce by flecainide include:

    I. Decreased duration of action potential
    II. Decreased rate of depolarization
    III. Constant action potential

    A. I only
    B. III only
    C. I and II only
    D. II and III only
    E. I, II, and III

184. Which of the following drugs are characterized by syncope on first dose?

    I. Captopril
    II. Pindolol
    III. Terazosin

    A. I only
    B. III only
    C. I and II only
    D. II and III only
    E. I, II, and III

185. All are side effects of loop diuretics therapy, EXCEPT:

    A. Decrease sodium
    B. Decrease potassium
    C. Decrease uric acid
    D. Decrease magnesium
    E. Decrease calcium

186. Which of the following drugs are preferred as antihypertensives for a pregnant patient?

   I. Methyldopa
  II. Hydralazine
 III. Enalapril

    A. I only
    B. III only
    C. I and II only
    D. II and III only
    E. I, II, and III

187. Domperidone is a:

    A. Serotonin antagonist
    B. Dopamine antagonist
    C. Serotonin agonist
    D. Dopamine agonist

Case Study: Questions 188 to 189

A 62 year old man with a history of Parkinson's disease has just received a prophylaxis against influenza A virus. The drug prescribed is also useful against Parkinson's disease.

188. Which of the following drugs has been prescribed?

   I. Amantadine
  II. Oseltamivir
 III. Zanamivir

    A. I only
    B. III only
    C. I and II only
    D. II and III only
    E. I, II, and III

189. What is the mechanism of the drug prescribed?

A. It prevents entry and penetration of the virus
B. It prevents uncoating of the virus
C. It prevents replication of the virus
D. It prevents release of the newly synthesized viruses
E. It prevents viral DNA replication

190. BT is admitted to the hospital with low blood pressure following overdose of chlorpromazine. An injection of epinephrine is given to restore his cardiovascular system, unfortunately the patient's condition did not show any sign of improvement. Which of the following statements is true regarding this observation?

A. Chlorpromazine depresses the respiratory center
B. Chlorpromazine is an adrenergic blocking agent
C. Chlorpromazine causes hypertension in toxic doses
D. Epinephrine decreases heart rate
E. Epinephrine is not effective in emergency situations

191. Mechanism of donezepil in the treatment of Alzheimer's disease:

A. Acetylcholine agonist
B. Acetylcholinesterase inhibitor
C. Acetylcholine reuptake inhibitor
D. Dopamine agonist
E. Dopamine reuptake inhibitor

192. Flumazenil is an antidote for:

A. Cholinergic drugs
B. Antidepressants
C. Opioids
D. Benzodiazepines
E. Salicylates

193. Vaginal yeast infection is characterized by:

A. Thick, white and clumpy discharge
B. Painful blisters in the genital area
C. Yellow pus like discharge
D. Gray cloudy discharge

194. Which of the following antidepressants has the highest degree of sedation?

A. Fluvoxamine
B. Citalopram
C. Moclobemide
D. Buproprion
E. Trazodone

195. Mechanism of action of glyburide:

A. Decreases glucose absorption
B. Increases insulin sensitivity
C. Increases insulin secretion
D. Decreases hepatic glucose production
E. Decreases insulin degradation

196. All of the following are class I antiarrhythmic drugs, EXCEPT:

A. Procainamide
B. Lidocaine
C. Quinidine
D. Propafenone
E. Amiodarone

197. All of the following are aminosteroids non-depolarizing neuromuscular blockers, EXCEPT:

A. Decamethonium
B. Pancuronium
C. Rocuronium
D. Vecuronium
E. Atracurium

198. All of the following are symptoms of atropine poisoning, EXCEPT:

A. Confusion
B. Blurred vision
C. Tachycardia
D. Miosis
E. Dizziness

199. Nausea caused by narcotics is due to:

A. Stimulation of adrenergic receptors
B. Inhibition of chemoreceptor trigger zone (CTZ) in brain
C. Inhibition of adrenergic receptors
D. Stimulation of chemoreceptor trigger zone (CTZ) in brain

200. Which of the following HIV drugs induces the formation of kidney stones?

A. Indinavir
B. Lopinavir
C. Nelfinavir
D. Ritonavir
E. Saquinavir

201. Mechanism of action of phenothiazines as antipsychotic drugs:

A. inhibition of muscarinic receptors
B. Inhibition of serotonin receptors
C. Inhibition of adrenergic receptors
D. Inhibiting of dopamine receptors
E. Inhibition of nicotinic receptors

202. Which of the following drugs acts as histamine receptor (H2) blocker?

A. Famotidine
B. Lansoprazole
C. Omeprazole
D. Amoxicillin
E. Misoprostol

203. All of the following substances produce and maintain general anesthesia by inhalation, EXCEPT:

A. Cyclopropane
B. Thiopental
C. Sevoflurane
D. Nitrous Oxide
E. Chloroform

204. Which of the following solution is required for the reconstitution of parenteral formulations?

A. USP Standard Highly Purified Water
B. USP Standard Sterile Water
C. USP Standard Water for Injection
D. USP Standard Purified Water for Injection
E. USP Standard Sterile Water for Injection

205. Which of the following vitamins is less likely to cause toxicity?

A. Vitamin E
B. Vitamin K
C. Vitamin A
D. Vitamin C
E. Vitamin D

206. Sumatriptan is an abortive treatment of migraines. Which of the following mechanisms applies to sumatriptan?

A. Serotonin agonist
B. Anticonvulsant
C. Beta blocker
D. Calcium channel blocker
E. Tricyclic antidepressant

207. Which of the following drugs is used to treat an acute asthma attack?

A. Theophylline
B. Montelukast
C. Salbutamol
D. Zafirlukast
E. Cromolyn

208. The following biological effects may be signs of anticholinergic drug therapy, EXCEPT:

A. Double vision (diplopia)
B. Loss of coordination (ataxia)
C. Diarrhea
D. Urinary retention
E. Xerostomia (dry mouth)

209. Which of the following drug categories is CONTRAINDICATED in women who are or may become pregnant?

A. Category D
B. Category B
C. Category C
D. Category X

210. Mechanism of action of trimethoprim:

A. Inhibits protein synthesis
B. Inhibits transcription
C. Dihydrofolate reductase inhibitor
D. DNA polymerase inhibitor
E. DNA ligase inhibitor

211. Transgenic animals can be produced by:

I. Stem cells mediated gene transfer
II. DNA microinjection
III. Retrovirus mediated gene transfer

    A. I only
    B. III only
    C. I and II only
    D. II and III only
    E. I, II, and III

212. Which of the following is NOT a cloning vector?

I. Mammalian cells
II. Bacterial artificial chromosomes (BACs)
III. Plasmid

    A. I only
    B. III only
    C. I and II only
    D. II and III only
    E. I, II, and III

213. Site-directed mutagenesis is a biotechnology technique useful in:

I. The production of mutant genes
II. Replacing individual amino acids in a protein sequence
III. The production of recombinant DNA

A. I only
B. III only
C. I and II only
D. II and III only
E. I, II, and III

214. Which of the following agents have the ability to decrease interfacial tension?

   I. Emulsifier
  II. Wetting agent
 III. Solubizer

    A. I only
    B. III only
    C. I and II only
    D. II and III only
    E. I, II, and III

215. Which of the following statements are true regarding thixotropy?

   I. Thixotrotic gels become fluidic when agitated
  II. The viscosity of thixotropic gels increases under pressure
 III. The viscosity of thixotropic gels increases by increasing shear rate

    A. I only
    B. III only
    C. I and II only
    D. II and III only
    E. I, II, and III

216. Which of the following statements are true regarding a plasmid?

   I. Used in biotechnology to produce DNA from RNA
  II. Circular DNA with self-replication capability
 III. Carry usually an antibiotic resistant gene

A. I only
B. III only
C. I and II only
D. II and III only
E. I, II, and III

217. Protein A has a binding site for ligand X with a Kd of 10^{-6} M. Protein B has a binding site for ligand X with a Kd of 10^{-9} M. Which of the following statements are true concerning proteins A and B?

A. Protein A has higher binding affinity for ligand X
B. Protein B has higher binding affinity for ligand X
C. Kd does not reflect binding affinity
D. Ka is more indicative of binding affinity
E. Inconclusive due to lack of information

Answers

1. B
The interaction is due to cimetidine inhibitory effect on CYP3A4. Rifampin, carbamazepine and phenytoin are inducers of CYP3A4 therefore they will enhance the metabolism of benzodiazepines. Statins, calcium channel blockers, azole antifungals, oral contraceptives, warfarin, antipsychotics, opiate analgesics, SSRIs, macrolides, chemothepapeutics and TCAs are other substrates of CYP3A4.

2. E

3. E
They decrease the threshold of seizures.

4. D
One of the side effects of antipsychotics is Parkinson's like syndrome.

5. E
The remaining drugs listed induce nausea and vomiting.

6. B

7. E

8. D

9. C
Cholestasis is a condition in which there is blockage of the flow of bile from liver to duodenum. Other drugs leading to cholestasis include cimetidine, estradiol, penicillin-based antibiotics, anabolic steroids, erythromycin, gold salts, imipramine, nitrofurantoin, oral contraceptives, prochlorperazine, sulindac and terbinafine.

10. D

Benzodiazepines and barbiturates enhance the brain inhibitory effect of gamma amino butyric acid (GABA).

11. D

12. E

Norepinephrine and acetycholine are also CNS neurotransmitters.

13. B

14. C

Presence of hydroxyl groups in 3 and 5 positions of the benzene ring increases resistance to catachol-O-methyl transferase (COMT) degradation and provides selectivity for beta 2 receptor.

15. D

Neostigmine is a positively charged ion (contains a quaternary amine) therefore is cannot cross the blood brain barrier unlike physostigmine which is uncharged.

16. D

17. B

Physostigmine or pilocarpine is antidote to scopolamine or atropine poisoning.

18. D

19. D

20. C

Common side effects are hypomagnesemia, hypocalcemia, hyperuricemia, leukopenia and thrombocytopenia.

21. E

22. B

23. E
Somatostatin, bromocriptine and corticosteroids have inhibitory effect on the release of growth hormone.

24. C

25. E

26. E

27. E

28. C
Omeprazole is a proton pump inhibitor. All the drugs listed are used in the treatment of ulcer. Ranitidine is a histamine-2 (H2) receptor blocker; aluminium hydroxide is an antacid; misoprostol inhibits adenylate cyclase in parietal cells resulting in decreased production of gastric acid; sucralfate neutralizes gastric acid.

29. A
Fluoxetine is a selective serotonin reuptake inhibitor (SSRI); trazodone is a serotonin reuptake inhibitor; bupropion is a dopamine reuptake inhibitor; methyphenydate is a psychostimulant.

30. A

31. C
Tyramine interacts with MAO inhibitors resulting in hypertensive crisis. Tyramine is also found in red wine and dark chocolate.

32. D

33. A
ACE Inhibitors prolong life. Aldosterone plays a role in worsening heart failure, and the remaining drugs have not been shown to prolong life in congestive heart failure. However, beta blockers and aldosterone antagonists (spironolactone) do prolong life in congestive heart failure.

34. B
Beta blockers lower cardiac output by blocking cardiac beta receptors and peripheral resistance is lowered by their effects on renin release. ACE inhibitors, alpha-1 blockers lower peripheral vascular resistance without reducing cardiac output.

35. B

36. C
Indapamide is a thiazide diuretic

37. C

38. C
A drug known to produce lupus-like syndrome is hydralazine. Bradycardia is incorrect since hydralazine produces tachycardia; cough is a side effect of ACE inhibitors; hypertrichosis is a side effect of minoxidil; hypokalemia is a side effect of thiazide diuretics.

39. E
The drug is a digitalis glycoside. Slowed AV (atrioventricular) node conduction is due to the action of digitalis in the brain, causing an activation of vagal tone to hyperpolarize the AV node, sometimes causing heart block. The antiarrhythmic properties result for the drug effect on the AV node. Increased myocardial contraction is due the direct effect of the drug on cardiac muscle.

40. E
Bretylium, ibutilide and sotalol are other potassium channel blockers. Sotalol is also a beta blocker.

41. E
Montelukast and zafirlukast are also leukotriene modifiers.

42. C
The patient has reflex tachycardia. When blood pressure decreases, the heart beats faster in an attempt to raise it, this effect is called reflex tachycardia. Methyldopa, propranolol and verapamil cause bradycardia. Minoxidil is not given as monotherapy.

43. E
Propranolol inhibits renin release, and thus lowers the concentrations of angiotensins I and II, and aldosterone. Captopril inhibits ACE, which lowers angiotensin II and aldosterone concentrations but increases angiotensin I concentration due to a loss of feedback inhibition of renin by angiotensin II. Losartan blocks angiotensin receptors and thus lowers aldosterone but increases the concentration of angiotensins I and II. Digoxin and nifedipine have insignificant effects on these substances.

44. D

45. C
Probenecid is called uricosuric drug. Sulfinpyrazone and allopurinol are also uricosuric drugs.

46. C
Fentany has the highest potency.

47. D

48. B

49. C
Target organ dysfunction is said to occur when there is retinopathy, nephropathy, cerebral or coronary insufficiency.

50. A
Afterload is best reflected by systemic vascular resistance. Preload is volume overload. Myocardial oxygen consumption is a reflection of the workload of the

heart and is estimated by heart rate and systolic blood pressure or it can be directly measured by gas exchange methods.

51. D
Methysergide, a serotonin blocker, is used for prevention.

52. C

53. B

54. E

55. E

56. D
Diuretics lead to increased levels of uric acid.

57. B

58. B
The best way to prevent this is to have a nitrate free period each day. If a patient is using a transdermal patch, removing it at night will provide a nitrate free period and reduce the risk of tolerance. Down regulation of receptors is usually seen with beta blockers. The combination of nitrates and sildenafil will result in profound drop in blood pressure (hypotension) due to synergistic effect.

59. D
Metformin is not associated with weight gain therefore it is preferred for obese diabetic patients. Standard dosage of metformin: 500 – 2500 mg daily. Start slow to minimize GI effects.

60. E

61. B

62. C
Rimantadine is used to treat influenza A infection.

63. E

64. E

65. B

66. D
Methadone is an agonist.

67. B
Morphine binds primarily to mu opioid receptors. Pupil dilation also called
mydriasis.

68. E
Pancytopenia is a reduction in red and white blood cells.

69. C
Codeine and dextromethorphan are other cough suppressants.

70. A
Doxycycline, minocycline, tetracycline are used orally. Erythromycin is used
orally or topically.

71. E

To prevent the irritation of the lining of esophagus, take with full glass of water
and avoid lying down for at least 30 minutes.

72. C

73. A

74. E

75. A
Imipenem is classified as carbapenem. Cephems are cephalosporins.

76. C
Other bactericidal drugs include penicillins and fluoroquinolones. Bacteriostatic drugs include tetracyclines, sulfonamides, macrolides and lincosamides.

77. B
8 to 12 hours drug-free period is required.

78. C
In gas chromatography the compounds to be separated must be volatile and stable at high temperature.

79. B
A chromophore contains electrons of low excitation energy. A molecule lacking a chromophore such as an aliphatic chain cannot absorb UV-Vis light.

80. C
Anion exchange occurs when the stationary phase is positively charged.

81. E

82. E

83. C
Sublingual tablets have the highest disintegration rate.

84. B

85. E
Osmotic pressure is another colligative property.

86. A
90% of the drug will be ionized therefore 100% - 90% = 10% unionized.
For an acidic drug, %ionized = 100 / 1 + antilog (pKa – pH); for a basic drug,
%ionized = 100 / 1 + antilog (pH – pKa)

87. D

88. A
A chiral centre is a carbon linked to four different groups. This molecules has $2^2 =$
4 possible isomers.

89. B

90. E
The binding of carbon monoxide (CO) to hemoglobin results in the formation of
carboxyhemoglobin and is the basis of CO poisoning. Oxygen administration is
an antidote.

91. A
The Michealis-Menten equation describes enzyme kinetics. K_m is the
concentration of substrate needed to reach half maximum velocity (V_{max})

92. E
A – D apply to regular tablet coating.

93. A

94. D
Gene expression is commonly regulated by hormones.

95. C
Their production is tedious which explains their high cost. Flu-like symptoms are common side effects of biotechnology drugs.

96. D

97. B
m/z is a measure of the molecular mass.

98. C

99. E
Basic drugs are more likely to bind to alpha 1-acid glycoprotein.

100. D

101 . C
C_0=Dose/Vd. Therefore C_0=500mg/(50kg x 2L/kg), 500 mg/100 L or 5 mg/L. Convert mg/L to ug/ml.

102 . B
90% of steady state will be reached in 3.3 half-lifes or 3.3 x 3.5 hours = 11.5 hours.

103. C
The relevant equation is: plasma drug concentration = Loading Dose or Dose / Vd.

104. B

105. D

106. C
Tendon rupture is a side effect of ciprofloxacin.

107. C

108. D

109. C

110. A
Titanium dioxide is also commonly found in sunscreen formulations.

111. E

112. D

113. B
Glycerides are also used as suppository base.

114. B

115. A
Cold cream is water in oil base; polyethylene glycol is water soluble base; lanolin is an absorption base.

116. D

117. A

118. B
Ephedrine is basic therefore it will become ionic in acidic environment which will enhance its water solubility.

119. B

120. C
Assuming they have the same elimination rate, the higher absorption rate will result in fastest onset of action.

121. D

122. A
Plasma pH = 7.4
Since pentobarbital is acidic the formula is:
% ionized = 100 / 1 + antilog (pka – pH)

123. C

124. B
Note: Priority assignment follows the atomic number.
I > Br > Cl > S > O > N > C > H

125. A
Note: Priority assignment follows the atomic number.
I > Br > Cl > S > O > N > C > H

126. A
Note: Priority assignment follows the atomic number.
I > Br > Cl > S > O > N > C > H

127. B
Note: Priority assignment follows the atomic number.
I > Br > Cl > S > O > N > C > H

128. B
Note: Priority assignment follows the atomic number.
I > Br > Cl > S > O > N > C > H

129. A
Note: Priority assignment follows the atomic number.
I > Br > Cl > S > O > N > C > H

130. B
Note: Priority assignment follows the atomic number.
I > Br > Cl > S > O > N > C > H

131. C

132. B

133. A

134. B

135. E

136. B
Other phase II reactions include methylation, sulfation, glucoronic acid conjugation, amino acid conjugation and glutathione conjugation.

137. A
Use the formula: Volume of distribution = Drug dosage / Drug concentration in plasma

138. B
Use the formula: Half life = 0.693 / Elimination rate

139. B
Use the formula: Half life = (0.693 x Volume of distribution) / Clearance

140. A

141. E
12 hours = 3 half lives; after 1 half life 400 mg /2 = 200 mg remains, after 2 half lives 200 mg /2 =100 mg remains, after 3 half lives 100 mg/2 = 50 mg remains.

142. A
Fick's for drug diffusion; Stoke's for sedimentation; Raoult's for vapor pressure; Poiseuille's for blood pressure (blood vessels resistance).

143. E

144. B

145. B
It is important to note that increasing the substrate concentration leads to the reversal of inhibition in competitive inhibition (curve 2); curve 1- no inhibitor; curve 3 – non competitive inhibition; curve 4 – mixed inhibition, mixed inhibition is more effective resulting in the highest decrease in reaction velocity.

146. B

147. C
The complementary sequence of DNA binds the first strand by complementary base pairing: A – T and C –G.

148. C
tRNA stands for transfer RNA

149. B

150. D

151. C

152. B

153. A

154. D

155. D
The target range of INR is higher for patients using warfarin; it is usually 2 to 3.

156. C
TDM is primarily required when a drug has narrow therapeutic index

157. E

158. B
PKU stands for phenylketonuria.

159. B
Forbe's disease is characterized by ineffective metabolism of carbohydrates.

160. C

161. B
Turbidity is a sign of bacterial meningitis.

162. D
Creatine kinase is a biomarker for myocardial infarction and muscles diseases.

163. E
Hexokinase is a biomarker for liver cancer.

164. C
Bromophenol blue test detects proteins.

165. A

166. A

167. C

168. C
Mercapturic acid is the end product of this reaction.

169. B

170. D
Serum creatinine is also needed.

171. A
Stomatitis is an inflammation of the lining of the mouth.

172. B

173. C
Secondary Raynaud's phenomenon may be caused by the following drugs: antineoplastics, cyclosporine, beta blockers, ergot derivatives and interferons.

174. C
Other antiemetic drugs used in the management of chemotherapy induced nausea and vomiting are metoclopramide, prochlorperazine, apprepitant, scopolamine, dimenhydrinate, haloperidol, benzodiazepines, serotonin antagonists, corticosteroids and opioids.

175. A
The remaining drugs listed are other useful alternatives.

176. D

177. E

178. D
As example, mannitol is an osmotic diuretic.

179. D
Other selective beta 1 blockers include betaxalol and bisoprolol; other non selective beta blockers include carteolol, carvedilol, labetalol, pindolol, sotalol, propranolol and timolol

180. D
Carvedilol has alpha blocking activity as well.
Oxprenolol has also intrinsic sympathomimetic activity. Beta blockers with intrinsic sympathomimetic activity (ISA) have agonistic and antagonistic effects, they act as partial agonists.

181. E
Antimuscarinics such as tolterodine; alpha blockers doxazosin, tamsulsoin and terazosin; 5-alpha reductase inhibitors such as finasteride and dutasteride.

182. D

183. D
Flecainide is a class IC antiarrhythmic.

184. B
First dose syncope is a characteristic of alpha blockers.

185. C

186. C

187. B
Domperidone is a peripheral dopamine antagonist.

188. A

189. A

190. B
As an adrenergic blocking agent chlorpromazine antagonizes the effect of epinephrine which explains its lack of effectiveness in this case. Chlorpromazine works on a variety of receptors in the central nervous system, producing anticholinergic, antidopaminergic, antihistaminic, and antiadrenergic effects.

191. B
The result is increased level of acetycholine and enhancement of cognition.

192. D

193. A
B refers to genital herpes, C refers to chlamydial infection and D refers to bacterial vaginosis.

194. E

195. C
Standard dosage of glyburide: 2.5 mg – 20 mg daily; give once daily up to 10 mg/day or in 2 divided doses if higher than 10 mg/day.

196. E
Amiodarone is a class III antiarrhythmic. Class I antiarrhythmics block sodium channel, class II are beta blockers (propranolol, esmolol, timolol), class III are potassium channel blockers (amiodarone, ibutilide) and class IV are calcium channel blockers (verapamil, diltiazem).

197. A
Decamethonium and succinylcholine are depolarizing neuromuscular blockers.

198. D
Mydriasis (pupil dilation) is one of the symptoms.

199. D

200. A
They all act as HIV protease inhibitors.

201. D
They inhibit primarily D2 receptor.

202. A
The drugs listed are all used to treat peptic ulcer however only antibiotic therapy (e.g. amoxicillin) is effective when ulcer is caused by H. Pylori infection. Other H2 receptor antagonists include cimetidine, ranitidine and nizatidine.

203. B
Thiopental is a short acting barbiturate and a non volatile anesthetic.

204. E
USP stands for United States Pharmacopeia.

205. D
Vitamin C is water soluble therefore it is cleared easily from the body compared to lipid soluble vitamins which have the tendency to accumulate in tissues.

206. A
Adverse effects of sumatriptan include flushing, dizziness, nausea and spasm of esophagus.

207. C

208. C
Anticholinergic drugs antagonize normal biological functions of cholinergic system. Therefore their effects are opposite to cholinergic system. Other adverse effects of anticholinergic drugs include mydriasis, constipation, increased body temperature, and tachycardia.

209. D
Category D is used only in serious or life-threatening situations.

210. C
Trimethoprim is a bacteriostatic antibiotic used mainly in prophylaxis and treatment of urinary tract infections; it is given commonly in combination with sulfamethoxazole, a sulfonamide.

211. E

212. A
Yeast artificial chromosome (YAC) is another type of cloning vector.

213. C

214. E

215. A
III describes a shear thinning gel. Synovial fluid found in joints is an example of thixotropic fluid. II describes an anthixotropic gel.

216. D
A plasmid requires a host such as bacteria for replication; a plasmid is used in biotechnology to introduce a foreign gene in bacteria.

217. B

PHARMACY PRACTICE

Questions

1. Which of the following drugs are used in the management of smoking cessation?

   I.   Clonidine
   II. Nortriptyline
   III. Varenicline

      A. I only
      B. III only
      C. I and II only
      D. II and III only
      E. I, II, and III

2. The following statements are correct regarding the drug raloxifene, EXCEPT:

      A. Used to manage post-menopausal symptom
      B. Used to treat and prevent ostoporosis.
      C. Decreases the risk of breast cancer
      D. Decreases HDL
      E. Increases hot flashes

3. Which of the following conditions may be worsen by heparin therapy?

      A. Liver insufficiency
      B. Kidney failure
      C. Hemolytic anemia
      D. Thrombocytopenia
      E. Biliary duct obstruction

4. Which of the following statements are true concerning terazosin?

   I.   May cause syncope.
   II. May cause fluid retention
   III. Use to treat benign prostate hyperplasia (BPH)

A. I only
B. III only
C. I and II only
D. II and III only
E. I, II, and III

5. Which of the following information is NOT included on the label of coal tar?

A. May cause photosensitivity
B. May stain cloth
C. Not effective in the treatment of head lice
D. Used to treat psoriasis
E. Is keratolytic

6. Carvedilol may produce which of the following effects?

I. Edema
II. Dizziness
III. Tachycardia

A. I only
B. III only
C. I and II only
D. II and III only
E. I, II, and III

7. All are correct statements regarding smoking cessation, EXCEPT.

A. Nicotine replacement is used to manage withdrawal symptoms
B. Nicotine patch may cause skin irritation at the site of application
C. Varenicline is used to decrease cravings
D. Nicotine patch can be used prior to stop day
E. Bupropion is used to decrease cravings

8. Septic shock is associated with the use of:

    I. Diaphragm
    II. Cervical cap
    III. Condom

        A. I only
        B. III only
        C. I and II only
        D. II and III only
        E. I, II, and III

9. Scabies in children is best treated with:

    I. Lindane
    II. 5% permethrin
    III. Crotamiton

        A. I only
        B. III only
        C. I and II only
        D. II and III only
        E. I, II, and III

10. Which of the following antihypertensives would you recommend to a patient of African descent?

    A. Propranolol
    B. Diltiazem
    C. Captopril
    D. Losartan
    E. Prazosin

11. Which of the following references would be best for locating the instructions for making a buffer for eye drop?

    I. Martindale extra pharmacopeia
    II. Remington
    III. Merck manual

A. I only
B. III only
C. I and II only
D. II and III only
E. I, II, and III

12. Which of the following is the drug of choice for the treatment of S.aureus infection?

A. Penicillin
B. Clindamycin
C. Erythromycin
D. Metronidazole
E. Vancomycin

13. Which of the following fungal drugs are not used topically?

I. Griseofulvin
II. Amphotericin B
III. Terbinafine

A. I only
B. III only
C. I and II only
D. II and III only
E. I, II, and III

14. GT is a patient on dialysis. He needs an antibiotic for the treatment of a minor infection. Which of the following antibiotics may exacerbate his chronic renal failure?

I. Doxycycline
II. Azithromycin
III. Cefaclor

A. I only
B. III only
C. I and II only
D. II and III only
E. I, II, and III

15. Which of the following antibiotics is the drug of choice for the treatment of methicillin-resistant Staphylococcus aureus (MRSA) infection?

    A. Linezolid
    B. Co-trimoxazole
    C. Clindamycin
    D. Doxycycline
    E. Vancomycin

16. Which of the following populations are at risk for the development of MRSA?

    I. Diabetics
   II. HIV patients
  III. Patients treated with quinolones

    A. I only
    B. III only
    C. I and II only
    D. II and III only
    E. I, II, and III

17. Which of the following is the best reference for foreign therapeutics?

    A. Martindale
    B. Compendium of Pharmaceuticals and Specialties (CPS)
    C. Therapeutic Choices
    D. Canadian Pharmacy Journal
    E. Compendium of Self-Care Products

18. Levodopa may produce all of the following biological effects, EXCEPT:

    A. Hallucinations
    B. Depression
    C. Nystagmus
    D. Confusion
    E. Hair loss (alopecia)

19. A18 yr. old girl is using oral contraceptives. Following sun exposure she has developed a brown rash. Which of the following may explain her condition?

   I. Acne or worsening of acne
  II. Sunburn
 III. Chloasma

    A. I only
    B. III only
    C. I and II only
    D. II and III only
    E. I, II, and III

20. A new medication has been just introduced on market. Which of the following parameters may determine having the medication in your pharmacy inventory?

   I. Cost of the medication
  II. Local use
 III. Side effects of the medication

    A. I only
    B. III only
    C. I and II only
    D. II and III only
    E. I, II, and III

21. Statins are effective lipid lowering drugs that decrease the production of cholesterol. Statins are taken once daily with the exception of:

  A. Rosuvastatin
  B. Fluvastatin
  C. Lovastatin
  D. Pravastatin
  E. Atorvastatin

22. You have just dispensed hydrochlorothiazide 50 mg BID for the treatment of edema. Which of the following information will NOT be provided to the patient?

    A. May increase body potassium level
    B. Avoid sun exposure
    C. Take in the morning
    D. Take with food to reduce GI upset
    E. Adverse effect include hyperuricemia, hyperglycemia and yellow vision

23. A patient with schizophrenia is complaining about extrapyramidal reactions such as restlessness and tremor. Which of the following drugs may be a good alternative?

    A. Risperidone
    B. Chlorpromazine
    C. Loxapine
    D. Fluphenazine
    E. Thiothixene

Case study: Questions 24 to 25

You are dispensing 500 mg SR tablets of sulfasalazine for the treatment of rheumatoid arthritis (RA).

24. Which of the following statements is NOT correct regarding sulfasalazine?

    A. Converted to sulfapyridine and 5-aminosalicylic acid (5-ASA) by intestinal flora
    B. Take after meal to provide longer transit time
    C. May change the color of urine
    D. Leads to agranulocytosis
    E. Sulfapyridine has anti-inflammatory effect

25. Which of the following conditions are treated with sulfasalazine?

    I. Ulcerative colitis
    II. Crohn's disease
    III. Scleroderma

A. I only
B. III only
C. I and II only
D. II and III only
E. I, II, and III

26. Which of the following drugs may NOT cause secondary dyslipidemia?

A. Thiazide diuretics
B. ACE inhibitors
C. Oral contraceptives
D. Antiretrovirals
E. Corticosteroids

27. Which of the following antibacterial drugs may cause photosensitivity?

I. Clindamycin
II. Erythromycin
III. Tetracycline

A. I only
B. III only
C. I and II only
D. II and III only
E. I, II, and III

28. The following statements are correct regarding atorvastatin, EXCEPT:

A. Interacts with azole antifungals
B. Decreases the production of cholesterol due to inhibition of HMG-CoA enzyme
C. Monitor liver enzymes during therapy
D. CYP3A4 inhibitors increase the toxicity of lovastatin
E. Taken in the morning

PR is a 65 year old patient. He is currently taking phenytoin 100 mg BID for 2 years. PR has just received a prescription for a statin to decrease his blood cholesterol.

29. The following statements are true regarding phenytoin, EXCEPT:

A. Phenytoin blocks voltage-sensitive sodium channels in neurons resulting in increased seizures threshold
B. Effective in the treatment of arrhythmias associated with QT prolongation
C. Effective in the treatment of trigeminal neuralgia (tic douloureux)
D. Effective in the treatment of absence seizures
E. Carbonic anhydrase inhibitors increase the toxicity of phenytoin

30. Which of the following statins would be appropriate for PR?

A. Atorvastatin
B. Lovastatin
C. Rosuvastatin
D. Pravastatin
E. Simvastatin

31. Which of the following antihypertensive drugs may be used in the management of alcohol withdrawal symptoms?

A. Clonidine
B. Propranolol
C. Captopril
D. Losartan
E. Hydrochlorothiazide

32. Ms. Young is complaining about heartburn and abdominal pain. Her profile shows that she is already taking ranitidine 150 mg BID for 5 weeks. Which of the following conditions may be your primary concern?

I. Ulcer
II. Gas
III. H. pylori

A. I only
B. III only
C. I and II only
D. II and III only
E. I, II, and III

33. All of the following are correct statements regarding omeprazole, EXCEPT:

A. Proton pump inhibitor in parietal cells
B. Decreases the clearance of warfarin, phenytoin and diazepam
C. Increases the absorption of digoxin
D. Taken without regard to food
E. Taken before meals and capsule should not be crushed

34. The clearance of theophylline is increased by all, EXCEPT:

A. Smoking
B. Carbamazepine
C. Ketoconazole
D. Rifampin
E. Age 1 to 9 years

35. A patient taking tylenol #3 is using docusate PO 200 mg to relief his constipation. Which of the following alternative may be suggested for enhanced effectiveness?

A. Take docusate and mineral oil
B. Take docusate and senna
C. Take docusate with methylcellulose
D. Stop docusate and start psyllium
E. Stop docusate and start senna

36. Cotrimoxazole auxiliary label may include all, EXCEPT:

A. May lead to allergic reactions
B. Photosensitivity is likely
C. Take with plenty of water
D. Maintain adequate fluid intake during therapy
E. Refrigerate the suspension after opening

37. All of the following are drugs used in the treatment of partial seizures, EXCEPT.

A. Gabapentin
B. Ethosuximide
C. Carbamazepine
D. Phenytoin
E. Topiramate

38. An obsessive compulsive patient taking fluoxetine is complaining about sexual dysfunction. Which of the following drugs may be a good alternative?

A. Nortriptyline
B. Mirtazapine
C. Sertraline
D. Citalopram
E. Clomipramine

39. Correct statements concerning the enzyme alteplase also known as tissue plasminogen activator.

I. Given orally
II. Clinical applications include pulmonary embolism, myocardial infarction and stroke
III. Enhances blood clot degradation via the conversion of plasminogen to plasmin

A. I only
B. III only
C. I and II only
D. II and III only
E. I, II, and III

40. Identify the first-line treatment for rheumatoid arthritis:

    A. Sulfasalazine
    B. Hydroxychloroquine
    C. Azathioprine
    D. Methotrexate
    E. Cyclosporine

41. Which of the anticonvulsants may be appropriate for an obese patient?

    A. Phenytoin
    B. Valproic acid
    C. Topiramate
    D. Carbamazapine
    E. Lamotrigine

42. All of the following are side effects of cephalosporins, EXCEPT.

    A. +ve Coomb's test
    B. Rash
    C. Hypersensitivity
    D. Superinfection
    E. Seizures

43. Stage II acetaminophen poisoning symptoms include:

    I. Liver enzymes elevation
    II. Abdominal pain
    III. Vomiting

    A. I only
    B. III only
    C. I and II only
    D. II and III only
    E. I, II, and III

44. Which of the following drugs may be the cause of urine discoloration?

    I. Metronidazole
    II. Cimetidine
    III. Rifampin

    A. I only
    B. III only
    C. I and II only
    D. II and III only
    E. I, II, and III

45. Ms. PR is a 17-year-old who is complaining about skin rash. She wonders if she is having another flare up of her eczema. She has a history of penicillin allergy, eczema and seizures. Ms. PR is currently using betamethasone Cr 0.05% bid prn, ethinyl estradiol/levonorgestrel for 12 months and phenytoin for 3 weeks. What is the likely explanation for her rash?

    A. An acute flare up of her eczema
    B. A reaction to phenytoin
    C. A reaction to oral contraceptives
    D. A reaction to betamethasone
    E. An interaction between ethinyl estradiol/levonorgestrel and phenytoin

Case Study: Questions 46 to 49

KC is a 3 years old child suffering from high fever. He is also complaining about ear pain. Otitis media is suspected.

46. Which of the following microorganisms cause otitis media?
    I. Streptococcus pneumoniae
    II. Haemophilus influenzae
    III. Moraxella catarrhalis

    A. I only
    B. III only
    C. I and II only
    D. II and III only
    E. I, II, and III

47. The drug of choice for the treatment of otitis media is:

A. Amoxicillin
B. Kanamycin
C. Penicillin
D. Cefaclor
E. Tetracycline

48. Which of the following are risk factors for the development of amoxicillin resistance in children?

I. Daycare attendance
II. Recent episode of otitis media
III. Recent antibiotic use

A. I only
B. III only
C. I and II only
D. II and III only
E. I, II, and III

49. In case of amoxicillin resistance which of the following drugs is commonly added to amoxicillin to enhance its effectiveness?

A. Ceftriaxone
B. Azithromycin
C. Clarithromycin
D. Clavulanate
E. Cefprozil

50. JO is a patient with treatment-resistant schizophrenia. He is also showing signs of suicidal behaviour. Which of the following medications would be the drug of choice for his treatment?

A. Olanzepine
B. Loxapine
C. Clozapine
D. Haloperidol
E. Thiothiene

51. Which of the following drugs causes metabolic acidosis?

I. Acetazolamide
II. Chlorthalidone
III. Furosemide

    A. I only
    B. III only
    C. I and II only
    D. II and III only
    E. I, II, and III

52. Which of the following statements are correct regarding the antihyperglycemic miglitol?

    I. Inhibits the enzyme alpha glucosidase
    II. Delays the digestion of carbohydrates
    III. Decreases postprandial hyperglycemia and levels of glycosylated hemoglobin

    A. I only
    B. III only
    C. I and II only
    D. II and III only
    E. I, II, and III

53. Urine glucose copper sulfate tests such as clinitest may be affected by:

    I. Isoniazid
    II. Levodopa
    III. Nalidixic acid

    A. I only
    B. III only
    C. I and II only
    D. II and III only
    E. I, II, and III

54. Potassium iodide label may include:

    I. Used as expectorant
    II. Stains
    III. External use only

    A. I only
    B. III only
    C. I and II only
    D. II and III only
    E. I, II, and III

55. Correct statement regarding warfarin-cotrimoxazole interaction.

    A. Trimethoprim decreases warfarin level
    B. Trimethoprim has no effect on warfarin level
    C. Sulfamethoxazole increases warfarin level
    D. Sulfamethoxazole has no effect on warfarin level
    E. Both sulfamethoxazole and trimethoprim decrease warfarin level

56. You are dispensing nifedipine 20 mg TID for the treatment of Prinzmental's angina (variant angina). The following information may be included in your counseling, EXCEPT:

    A. Keep in amber glass of bottle
    B. Adverse effects include facial flushing, dizziness, peripheral edema and heat sensitivity
    C. Take without regard to grapefruit juice
    D. Increases digoxin toxicity
    E. Cimetidine increases nifedipine toxicity

57. A patient has a non productive cough. Which of the following may be of concern?

    I. Antihypertensive therapy
    II. Asthma
    III. Smoking

A. I only
B. III only
C. I and II only
D. II and III only
E. I, II, and III

58. You are counseling an asthmatic patient regarding the proper use of Diskus. Diskus is a dry powder inhaler that holds 60 doses. Which of the following statements will NOT be included in your counseling?

A. Slide the lever away to load your medication.
B. Close mouth around the mouth piece
C. Dose ready to take
D. Hold breath for 10 seconds then breath out
   Always check the dose counter

59. Side effects of accutane include all, EXCEPT:

A. Urticaria
B. Conjunctivitis
C. Photosensitivity
D. Thinning of hair
E. Runny nose

60. Which of the following drugs is not used in the treatment of bacterial meningitis?

A. Chloramphenicol
B. Ceftriaxone
C. Flucytosine
D. Vancomycin
E. Rifampin

61. Which of the following statements are correct regarding vitamin C?

I. It is a coenzyme
II. It is associated with the formation of kidney stones
III. It enhances the absorption of iron

A. I only
B. III only
C. I and II only
D. II and III only
E. I, II, and III

62. All of the following are correct statements concerning raloxifene, EXCEPT.

A. Given once daily with or without food
B. Has long duration of action, 24-48 hours
C. Decreases the risk of deep vein thrombosis
D. May increase hot flashes in postmenopausal women
E. Monitor liver function for long-term use

63. All of the following are risk factors for cardiovascular diseases, EXCEPT

A. Family history of cardiovascular diseases
B. Smoking
C. Menopause
D. Caucasian
E. Sedentary lifestyle

64. All of the following are risk factors for osteoporosis, EXCEPT

A. Smoking
B. Caucasian or Asian
C. Hyperthyroidism
D. Obesity
E. Corticosteroids therapy

65. Doxycycline label may include all, EXCEPT.

A. May discolor teeth
B. May induce sun sensitivity
C. Do not take with aluminum, magnesium, or calcium based antacids as their reduce doxycycline absorption
D. Not contraindicated during pregnancy
E. Phenytoin and carbamazepine reduce doxycycline bioavailability

66. Iron deficiency is characterized by:

   I. Increased serum ferritin
  II. Increase iron binding capacity
 III. Increased serum transferrin

     A. I only
     B. III only
     C. I and II only
     D. II and III only
     E. I, II, and III

67. Which of the following drugs are used for the treatment of bacterial conjunctivitis?

   I. Sulfacetamide
  II. Gatifloxacin
 III. Neomycin

     A. I only
     B. III only
     C. I and II only
     D. II and III only
     E. I, II, and III

68. Voltaren eye drop may produce which of the following side effects?

   I. Stinging and burning
  II. Irritation and redness
 III. Miosis

     A. I only
     B. III only
     C. I and II only
     D. II and III only
     E. I, II, and III

69. A 34 years old patient has been experiencing the following symptoms for the past few weeks: fatigue, constipation, cold intolerance and depression. Which of the following should be evaluated?

    A. Liver function
    B. Thyroid function
    C. Brain function
    D. Kidney function
    E. Heart function

70. Correct statements concerning zoplicone a non-benzodiazepine hypnotic:

    I. May increase falls in elderly
    II. Tolerance may develop after few weeks of therapy
    III. May be used to treat depression

        A. I only
        B. III only
        C. I and II only
        D. II and III only
        E. I, II, and III

71. Methotrexate may produce the following adverse effets, EXCEPT:

    A. Gingivitis
    B. Rash
    C. Hepatotoxicity
    D. Leukopenia
    E. Weight gain

72. Hormone replacement therapy (HRT) is contraindicated in the following conditions, EXCEPT:

    A. Coronary artery disease
    B. Hepatic disease
    C. Gallbladder disease
    D. Osteoporosis
    E. Unexplained vaginal bleeding

73. The benefits of hormone replacement therapy include all, EXCEPT:

A. Hot flashes
B. Night sweats
C. Sleep difficulties
D. Vaginal dryness
E. Decrease incidence of breast cancer

74. All of the following are risk factors for atopic dermatitis, EXCEPT:

A. Female
B. Family history of asthma
C. Exposure to skin irritants (e.g. wool, soaps, cosmetics, perfumes, dust, chemicals)
D. Use of moiturizers after bathing
E. Exposure to extreme temperature (cold or hot)

75. Diabetics morning increase in blood sugar could be managed by the administration of extra insulin in the evening. Other options include:

I. Change long-acting insulin administration time to late evening so that its peak action occurs when blood sugars start rising.
II. Switch to a longer acting insulin in the evening
III. Switch to insulin pump which can release additional insulin

A. I only
B. III only
C. I and II only
D. II and III only
E. I, II, and III

76. Which of the following statements is NOT correct regarding iron?

A. Can be given with milk
B. Causes constipation or diarrhea
C. Stomach acidity increases it's absorption
D. Most abundant metal in the body
E. It's deficiency is a common cause of anemia

77. Correct statements concerning horizontal flow hood:

   I. Does not protect operator
  II. Ensures maximum preparations sterility
 III. Could be used for carcinogenic preparations

     A. I only
     B. III only
     C. I and II only
     D. II and III only
     E. I, II, and III

78. Meta analysis is:

     A. Combination of several studies that address related research hypotheses
     B. Assessment of the similarity between means of more than two groups
     C. Assessment of the similarity between two means
     D. Evaluation of differences between two variances
     E. Study of the correlation between variables

79. Lugol's solution label may include all, EXCEPT:

     A. Store at room temperature
     B. Caution medication may stain
     C. Contains 35% alcohol
     D. Used as reagent in Chiller's test
     E. Used as disinfectant and antiseptic

80. A patient has brain tumor. Which of the following should not be part of the pharmacist's counseling?

     A. Discuss patient's new treatment regimen
     B. Disease evaluation
     C. Patient's profile updating
     D. Drug-drug interactions review
     E. Side effects review

81. All of the following are correct statements concerning sumatriptan, EXCEPT.

A. Is a selective serotonin receptor agonist
B. Is effective at any stage of headaches
C. Can take another tablet if there is no relief after 1 hour
D. Effective in the treatment of cluster headaches as well
E. Relieves photophobia, phonophobia, nausea and vomiting associated with migraine headache

82. A pharmacy manager wants to reduce errors of dispensing. He would invite all of following, EXCEPT.

A. Registered nurse
B. Patient
C. Senior pharmacist
D. Pharmacy technicians
E. Good practice manager

83. Identify the recommended therapeutic range of lithium:

A. 0.3 – 0.7 mEq/L
B. 0.8 – 1.2 mEq/L
C. 1.5 – 2.3 mEq/L
D. 2.5 mEq/L – 3.1 mEq/L
E. mEq/L – 3.9 mEq/L

84. Which of the following vaccines does not require refrigeration?

A. Flu
B. MMR
C. Pneumococcal
D. Chicken pox
E. Haemophilus influenzea B

85. Correct statements concerning the antimetabolite 5-fluorouracil cream:

I. Apply with a non-metallic applicator or fingertips
II. Topical treatment of skin cancer
III. Avoid sun exposure

A. I only
B. III only
C. I and II only
D. II and III only
E. I, II, and III

86. Which of the following cancer drugs are associated with high incidence of cardiotoxicity?

I. Doxorubicin
II. Mithoxantrone
III. Cyclophosphamide

A. I only
B. III only
C. I and II only
D. II and III only
E. I, II, and III

87. All of the following are correct statements concerning filgrastim, EXCEPT.

A. Used to treat neutropenia by stimulating the bone marrow to produce more neutrophils
B. Antagonizes the effects of immunosuppressants
C. Is a granulocyte colony-stimulating factor
D. Refrigerate. Discard if stored at room temperature longer than 6 hours
E. Associated with severe side effects

88. Which of the following statements are true regarding glyburide and glimepiride:

I. They have similar effect on fasting glucose and glycosylated hemoglobin level
II. There is lower incidence of hypoglycemia with glimepiride
III. They have similar duration of action

A. I only
B. III only
C. I and II only
D. II and III only
E. I, II, and III

89. Correct statements regarding infliximab:

    I. Immunomodulator and anti-inflammatory agent
    II. Used as DMARD
    III. Adverse effects include increased risk of opportunistic infections

    A. I only
    B. III only
    C. I and II only
    D. II and III only
    E. I, II, and III

90. All of the following are symptoms of child dehydration, EXCEPT.

    A. Sunken eyes
    B. Dry mouth
    C. Turgor skin
    D. Fever
    E. Increased heart rate

91. Identify the recommended therapeutic range of phenytoin:

    A. 5- 9 mcg/mL
    B. 10 – 20 mcg/mL
    C. 22 - 35 mcg/mL
    D. 40 – 57 mcg/mL
    E. 60 – 72 mcg/mL

92. Which of the following antibodies is used in the treatment of breast cancer?

    A. Infliximab
    B. Muromonab
    C. Abciximab
    D. Trastuzumab
    E. Adalimumab

93. Correct statements regarding typhoid vaccine:

A. Given at 2 months, 4 months, 6 months and 18 months
B. 3 injections at any age with the second and third shots respectively 1 and 6 months after the first
C. Single dose for people any age at risk such as travelers to areas with poor sanitation
D. Given at 12 months and 18 months

94. Pertussis (whooping cough) vaccine is given to children in combination with:

I. Diphtheria
II. Tetanus
III. Mumps

A. I only
B. III only
C. I and II only
D. II and III only
E. I, II, and III

95. Which of the following statements are correct regarding the biological effects of moclobemide?

I. Reversible inhibitor of MAO-A
II. Decreases the degradation of serotonin, norepinephrine and dopamine
III. Selective serotonin reuptake inhibitor

A. I only
B. III only
C. I and II only
D. II and III only
E. I, II, and III

96. PIPEDA stands for:

    A. Privacy Information Protection and Electronic Documents Agency
    B. Personal Information Policy and Electronic Documents Access
    C. Privacy Information Protection and Electronic Documents Access
    D. Privacy Information Policy and Electronic Documents Agency
    E. Personal Information Protection and Electronic Documents Act

97. Rx
Ephedrine HCl
Nacl.
Na bisulphite.
Na bisulphate is used as:

I. Chelating agent
II. Antimicrobial
III. Antioxidant.

    A. I only
    B. III only
    C. I and II only
    D. II and III only
    E. I, II, and III

98. Following an overdose of aspirin its clearance is enhanced by the administration of:

    A. Ammonium chloride
    B. Ascorbic acid
    C. Iron dextran
    D. Calcium chloride
    E. Sodium bicarbonate

99. The recommended daily dosage of clarithromycin for a child is 11.5 mg/kg. For a patient weighing 9.7 kg, calculate the amount of a 150mg/5mL suspension needed for one week treatment.

    A. 13.0 mL
    B. 26.0 mL
    C. 35.0 mL
    D. 41.0 mL
    E. 52.0 mL

100. A patient presents a prescription with the following antiviral drug regimen: start with 50 mg then decrease by 10 mg every 2 days until finished. How many 5 mg tablets are needed to fill this prescription?

A. 20
B. 40
C. 60
D. 80
E. 100

101. A vial of sodium chloride (NaCl) injection contains 3 mEq of sodium chloride per mL. What is the percentage strength of this solution? Molecular weight of sodium chloride is 58.44 g.

A. 9.0%
B. 13.2%
C. 17.5%
D. 21.6%
E. 30.0%

102. What is the required infusion rate (ml/min) to deliver the desired dose of 5ug/kg/min to a 75 kg patient within 6 hours. The infusion solution has a concentration of 400 ug/mL.

A. 0.50mL/min
B. 0.93 mL/min
C. 1.25 mL/min
D. 1.80 mL/min
E. 2.10 mL/min

103. Which of the following benzodiazepines has the longest duration of action?

A. Flurazepam
B. Alprazolam
C. Midazolam
D. Triazolam
E. Diazepam

104. Which of the following drugs are used mostly in the management of status epilepticus?

    I. Valproate
   II. Lorazepam
  III. Fosphenytoin

      A. I only
      B. III only
      C. I and II only
      D. II and III only
      E. I, II, and III

105. Drug of choice for petit mal:

A. Carbamazepine
B. Ethosuximide
C. Phenytoin
D. Lorazepam
E. Primidone

106. Indication of sulfinpyrazone:

A. Treatment of Parkinson's
B. Treatment of depression
C. Treatment of viral infections
D. Treatment of fungal infection
E. Treatment of gout

107. Which of the following antihypertensives are preferred for a diabetic patient?

    I. Torsemide
   II. Nadolol
  III. Captopril

      A. I only
      B. III only
      C. I and II only
      D. II and III only
      E. I, II, and III

108. Biological effects of lipid-lowering drug fenofibrate:

    I. Binds bile acids in the intestine to promote their excretion
    II. Inhibits the synthesis of cholesterol
    III. Increases the degradation of lipids and the removal of LDL from the bloodstream

    A. I only
    B. III only
    C. I and II only
    D. II and III only
    E. I, II, and III

109. Drug of choice for hyperthyroidism during pregnancy:

A. Carbimazole
B. Atenolol
C. Radioactive iodine
D. Propylthiouracil
E. Iodine

110. Mechanism of thionamides in the treatment of hyperthyroidism:

I. Destroy thyroid gland
II. Inhibit the effects of thyroid stimulating hormone
III. Decrease the production of thyroid hormone

    A. I only
    B. III only
    C. I and II only
    D. II and III only
    E. I, II, and III

111. Drug of choice for the prevention of blood coagulation during pregnancy:

    A. Heparin
    B. Aspirin
    C. Warfarin
    D. Ticlopidine
    E. Clopidrogel

112. All of the following are nucleoside reverse transcriptase inhibitors used to treat HIV infection, EXCEPT:

A. Abacavir
B. Stavudine
C. Didanosine
D. Nevirapine
E. Zidovudine

113. Which of the following conditions are complications of diabetes?

I. Atherosclerosis
II. Carpal tunnel syndrome
III. Impaired vision

A. I only
B. III only
C. I and II only
D. II and III only
E. I, II, and III

114. The following statements are true regarding lithium therapy, EXCEPT.

A. Recommended dosage in the range of 600 mg to 1200 mg per day
B. Use in the treatment of bipolar depression
C. Side effects include tremor, excessive thirst and urination, thyroid gland insufficiency and several gastrointestinal effects
D. Onset of action is usually from 2 – 3 weeks.
E. Therapeutic drug monitoring is not required due to narrow therapeutic index

115. Mechanism of action of the antidepressant paroxetine:

A. Inhibition of serotonin reuptake
B. Psychostimulation
C. Dopamine agonist
D. Monoamine oxidase inhibition
E. Inhibition of norepinephrine reuptake

116. Which of the following mechanisms applies to bimatoprost used to treat glaucoma?

A. Decrease aqueous humor production
B. Increase aqueous humor production
C. Increase aqueous humor outflow
D. Decrease aqueous humor outflow

117. The following drug classes are used to treat glaucoma, EXCEPT:

A. Prostaglandin-like drugs
B. Anticholinergic drugs
C. Carbonic anhydrase inhibitors
D. Alpha agonists
E. Beta blockers

118. Correct statements regarding dyskinesia:

I. Movement disorder characterized by diminished voluntary movements and the presence of involuntary movements
II. Tardive dyskinea results from treatment with an antipsychotic such as haloperidol
III. Vermicular tongue movement is the early sign of tardive dyskinesia

    A. I only
    B. III only
    C. I and II only
    D. II and III only
    E. I, II, and III

119. Combining levodopa to carbidopa is the highlight of treatment of Parkinson's disease because:

I. Carbidopa induces peripheral conversion of levodopa to dopamine
II. Carbidopa decreases dopamine side effects on the periphery
III. Carbidopa increase the concentration of levodopa and dopamine in the brain

A. I only
B. III only
C. I and II only
D. II and III only
E. I, II, and III

120. All of the following are side effects of MAO inhibitors, EXCEPT:

A. Insomnia.
B. Hypotension
C. Pins-and-needles sensation
D. Sexual dysfunction
E. Seizures

121. Long term use of hydrocortisone may produce all of the following effects, EXCEPT:

A. Sodium retention
B. Hypoglycemia
C. Hypercalcemia
D. Increased susceptibility to infection
E. Peptic ulceration.
F. Osteoporosis

122. Which one of the following agents is NOT keratolytic?

A. Salicylic acid
B. Urea
C. Lactic acid
D. Allantoin
E. Sulfur
F. Ascorbic acid

123. Vitamin A deficiency is primarily characterized by:

A. Bone thinning
B. Sore tongue
C. Night blindness
D. Bleeding gums
E. Tendency to bleed

124. Correct statements regarding edema:

   I. Accumulation of fluid beneath the skin or in body cavities
  II. Is caused by increased secretion of fluid into interstitial tissue or impaired removal of fluid
 III. May be a sign of heart failure

    A. I only
    B. III only
    C. I and II only
    D. II and III only
    E. I, II, and III

125. Gynecomastia is one of the side effects of spironolactone. Which of the following characterizes gynecomastia?

    A. Menstrual irregularities
    B. Painful menstruation
    C. Lack of menstruation
    D. Breast enlargement in men
    E. Sexual dysfunction in men

126. Which of the following calcium channel blockers (CCBs) causes constipation?

A. Nifidipine
B. Diltiazem
C. Verapamil
D. Nicardipine
E. Amlodipine

127. The following statements are correct regarding chronic hemochromatosis, EXCEPT:

   A. Secondary hemochromatosis can be caused by thalassemia
   B. Excessive deposition of iron in tissues leading to darkening of skin color
   C. May lead to hepatic cirrhosis and diabetes mellitus
   D. Low transferrin saturation is indicative of iron overload
   E. The goal of treatment is to remove excess iron from the body and treat any organ damage

128. Tapeworm infection is effectively treated with:

   I.   Praziquantel
   II. Niclosamide
   III. Ivermectin

      A. I only
      B. III only
      C. I and II only
      D. II and III only
      E. I, II, and III

129. All of the following statements are correct regarding necrosis, EXCEPT:

   A. Death of cells or tissues
   B. May be caused by naturally occurring cell death
   C. Caused by ischemia
   D. Caused by inflammation
   E. Caused by infection

130. Which of the following biomolecules antagonize the body inflammatory processes?

A. Prostaglandins
B. Leukotrienes
C. Histamine
D. Pyrogens
E. Steroids

131. Wrong statement regarding the difference between acute inflammation and chronic inflammation:

A. Acute inflammation is primarily mediated by granulocytes whereas chronic inflammation is primarily associated with the activity of monocytes and lymphocytes
B. Acute inflammation may lead to abscess formation and chronic inflammation
C. Chronic inflammation may lead to tissues destruction
D. The onset of acute inflammation is usually delayed
E. Chronic inflammation may be caused by autoimmune disorders

132. Cholecystitis is characterized by:

A. Inflammation of appendix
B. Inflammation of kidneys
C. Inflammation of colon
D. Inflammation of gall Bladder
E. Inflammation of liver

133. The following statements apply to losartan, EXCEPT:

A. Antihypertensive
B. Angiotensin II blocker
C. Beta blocker
D. Acts as a prodrug
E. Metabolized to produce a more potent 5-carboxylic acid derivative

134. Which of the following anthelmintics is effective in the treatment trematode infections?

A. Praziquantel
B. Pyrantel Pamoate
C. Ivermectin
D. Albendazole
E. Mebendazole

135. Correct statements regarding tinea pedis:

   I. Viral infection
  II. Fungal infection
 III. Over-the-counter treatments include 2% miconazole nitrate and 1% tolnaftate

    A. I only
    B. III only
    C. I and II only
    D. II and III only
    E. I, II, and III

136. Correct statements regarding malaria prophylaxis:

   I. Drug effect does not start immediately thus travelers should start taking their medications, in general, one or two weeks prior to visiting a malaria-endemic area
  II. Prophylatic drugs include mefloquine, doxycycline and the combination atovaquone/proguanil
 III. Travelers should discontinue treatment immediately after leaving a malaria-endemic area

    A. I only
    B. III only
    C. I and II only
    D. II and III only
    E. I, II, and III

137. Bismuth subsalicylate is an adsorbent used to treat diarrhea and may cause blackening of stool. Which of the following diarrhea treatment agents has the same mechanism of action?

A. Loperamide
B. Paregoric
C. Codeine
D. Tincture of opium
E. Kaolin

138. Correct statements regarding docusate:

   I. Stool softeners
  II. Use to treat and prevent constipation
 III. Flatulence is also a common side effect

     A. I only
     B. III only
     C. I and II only
     D. II and III only
     E. I, II, and III

139. All of the following are stimulant laxatives used to treat constipation, EXCEPT:

A. Bisacodyl
B. Senna
C. Castor oil
D. Sorbitol
E. Cascara

140. The clearance of theophylline is decreased by all, EXCEPT:

     A. Cimetidine
     B. Azithromycin
     C. Ciprofloxacin
     D. Oral contraceptives
     E. Fatty meals

141. A 45 years old patient is seeking counseling concerning a persistent vaginal irritation for the last 5 months. She has tried miconazole and clotrimazole 3 day therapy. Both were effective but the problem reoccurs. Her symptoms include frequent urination and thirst. She has not seen her physician for almost two years.

A likely explanation would be:

A. Diabetic and the sugar spilling into her urine may be causing a recurrent yeast infections
B. Diabetic but the yeast infections could not be associated with the sugar in her urine
C. Incorrect use of antifungal drug. Recurrent infections respond better to 6-day therapy
D. Overusing non-prescription antifungals and the subsequent bacterial overgrowth is contributing to her recurrent bacterial infections

142. Labeling of cotrimoxazole suspension may include:

I. Take with lot of liquid
II. Shake well before using
III. Exposure to sunlight may cause adverse reactions

    A. I only
    B. III only
    C. I and II only
    D. II and III only
    E. I, II, and III

143. Rx

Betaxolol 0.32% drops
Mitte: 10 mL
Sig: gtt. i o.u. TID

Which of the following instructions will be on the prescription label?

A. Apply one drop into both eyes three times per day
B. Apply one drop into the right eye three times per day
C. Apply one drop into the left eye two times per day
D. Apply one drop into both eyes two times per day
E. Apply one drop into the right eye two times per day

144. The following prescription is received in a hospital pharmacy:

Losartan 25 mg
S: Take 1 tab BID
M: 3 weeks

Which of the following instructions will be on the prescription label?

    A. Take one tablet once daily (21 tablets)
    B. Take two tablets once daily (42 tablets)
    C. Take one tablet twice daily (42 tablets)
    D. Take half tablet twice weekly (21 tablets)
    E. Take two tablets twice daily (48 tablets)

145. Which of the following drugs is used in an emergency room to treat cardiac arrest?

    I.   Nitroglycerine
    II. Diphenhydramine
    III. Epinephrine

        A. I only
        B. III only
        C. I and II only
        D. II and III only
        E. I, II, and III

146. Dry mouth is the side effect of which of the following asthma drugs?

A. Theophylline
B. Salbutamol
C. Ipratopium
D. Beclomethasone
E. Montelukast

147. Patients taking certain asthma drugs should be counsel on possible change of voice and fungal infection of the mouth (trush) as side effects. Which of the following drug classes is concerned?

A. Mast cell stabilizers
B. Corticosteroids
C. Leukotrienes modifiers
D. Anticholinergic
E. Beta agonists

148. Which of the following antibiotic classes can lead to hearing loss (ototoxicity)?

A. Cephalosporins
B. Macrolides
C. Aminoglycosides
D. Penicillins
E. Tetracyclines

149. Which of the following antibiotics have allergic reactions as side effects?

  I. Ceftazidime
 II. Nafcillin
III. Sulfacetamide

    A. I only
    B. III only
    C. I and II only
    D. II and III only
    E. I, II, and III

150. CPS (Compendium of Pharmaceuticals and Specialties) is a useful resource for finding:

  I. Drug monographs
 II. Drug identification chart
III. Clinical recommendations for dental prophylaxis of bacterial infection

A. I only
B. III only
C. I and II only
D. II and III only
E. I, II, and III

151. Identify the correct formulation of Tylenol #2:

A. 300 mg acetaminophen, 8 mg codeine, 15 mg caffeine
B. 300 mg acetaminophen, 30 mg codeine, 15 mg caffeine
C. 300 mg acetaminophen, 15 mg codeine, 15 mg caffeine
D. 300 mg acetaminophen, 60 mg codeine

152. Following an overdose of amphetamine its clearance may be enhanced by the administration of:

A. Potassium chloride
B. Ascorbic acid
C. Sodium chloride
D. Sodium bicarbonate
E. Calcium chloride

153. Which of the following abbreviations means "with meals"?

A. aa
B. pc
C. po
D. cc
E. cp

154. Which of the following abbreviations means "at bed time"?

A. pm
B. hs
C. hp
D. bt
E. bm

155. Appropriate information to provide to a patient regarding the use of beclomethasone inhaler includes:

   I.   Gargle and rinse your mouth after use
   II. Rinsing the mouth helps to prevent dryness, relieve throat irritation and to prevent oral yeast infections
   III. Shake the canister well before using

   A. I only
   B. III only
   C. I and II only
   D. II and III only
   E. I, II, and III

156. Which of the following statements is correct regarding the use of salicylates (NSAIDs) in the treatment of rheumatoid arthritis:

A. Analgesic and anti-inflammatory effects
B. Cure completely the disease
C. More effective than corticosteroids
D. More effective than immunosuppressive drugs
E. Decrease the progression of the disease

157. Which of the following medicinal herb increases the incidence of digoxin toxicity?

A. St. John's wort
B. Echinacea
C. Ginseng
D. Feverfew
E. Gingko

158. Which of the following conditions may prevent the use of theophylline in the treatment of asthma?

A. Peptic ulcer
B. Diabetes
C. Congestive heart failure
D. Young age
E. Smoking

159. Which of the following resources provide information on the selection of drug therapy regimen?

   I. Compendium of self-care
  II. Clinical guidelines publications
 III. Harrison's principles of internal medicine

     A. I only
     B. III only
     C. I and II only
     D. II and III only
     E. I, II, and III

160. Wrong statement regarding orlistat:

     A. Its primary function is the prevention of dietary fat absorption
     B. Its effectiveness increases with low fat diet
     C. It inhibits pancreatic lipase
     D. The primary side effects of the drug are gastrointestinal related such as steatorrhea
     E. It reduces the absorption of fat soluble vitamins

161. Appropriate information to provide to a patient regarding the administration of orlistat includes:

   I. Take during a meal
  II. Take up to one hour following a meal
 III. Take up to one hour before a meal

     A. I only
     B. III only
     C. I and II only
     D. II and III only
     E. I, II, and III

162. Emphysema is characterized by:

    I. Shortness of breath
   II. Enlargement of small sacs in lungs and damage of alveolar in lungs
  III. Alpha 1-antitrypsin deficiency

    A. I only
    B. III only
    C. I and II only
    D. II and III only
    E. I, II, and III

163. Which of the following medicinal herbs decreases the effectiveness of potassium-sparing diuretics?

A. Chamomile
B. Ginkgo
C. Licorice
D. Ginger
E. Saw Palmetto

164. Which of the following statements describes best SPF 30?

    A. Offers protection 30 times longer than if no sunscreen is used
    B. 30% (w/v) concentration of active substance
    C. 30% (w/v) concentration of formulation excipients
    D. Provides 30 minutes protection
    E. Apply 30 minutes prior to sun exposure

165. All of the following statements are correct regarding nicotine replacement therapy, EXCEPT:

    A. Nicotine replacement products include nicotine patch, nicotine pastilles/lozenges, nicotine gum and nicotine inhaler
    B. Each piece of nicotine gum typically contains 2 or 4 mg of nicotine roughly the nicotine content of 1 or 2 cigarettes
    C. A patch contains from 5 mg to 22 mg of nicotine
    D. Helps stop nicotine cravings and relieve withdrawal symptoms
    E. Start with low-dose patch then increase gradually

166. Rifampin may produce all the following effects, EXCEPT:

A. Rash
B. Seizures
C. Red-orange colored tears
D. Liver dysfunction
E. Thrombocytopenia

167. In general, what is the optimum storage temperature of biopharmaceuticals?

    A. - 80 °C
    B. - 15 °C
    C. 2- 8 °C
    D. A cool place
    E. Room temperature

168. How many grams of zinc oxide are needed to make 240 grams of 4% (w/w) zinc oxide ointment?

A. 12.0 g
B. 9.6 g
C. 7.8 g
D. 4.5 g
E. 2.0 g

169. How many milliliters of 1:50 stock solution of epinephrine HCl solution should be used to prepare one liter of 1:4000 solution?

A. 50 mL
B. 32.5 mL
C. 25 mL
D. 12.5 mL
E. 6.0 mL

170. A pharmacist has a 70% alcoholic elixir and a 20% alcoholic elixir. She needs a 30% elixir to use in the formulation of a drug. In what proportion must 70% elixir and 20% elixir be combined to make 30% elixir?

A. 1 part of 70% and 4 parts of 20%
B. 2 parts of 70% and 4 parts of 20%
C. 2 parts of 70% and 3 parts of 20%
D. 1 part of 70% and 5 parts of 20%
E. 1 part of 70% and 3 parts of 20%

171. The following strategies are appropriate for the prevention of allergic rhinitis, EXCEPT:

   A. Avoid dust and other triggers
   B. Opening windows to get fresh air
   C. Ensure a clean living environment
   D. Removal of all carpets
   E. Regular vacuuming

172. What is the meaning of the Latin abbreviation "ad lib"?

   A. as dispensed
   B. as directed
   C. as needed
   D. as desired
   E. as instructed

173. What is the meaning of the Latin abbreviation "qam"?

   A. Every hour
   B. Every week
   C. Every morning
   D. Every afternoon
   E. Every evening

174. What is the meaning of the pharmacy term "PR"?

A. Vaginally
B. Sublingual
C. Inhalation
D. Transdermal
E. Rectally

175. What is the meaning of the medical abbreviation "D5W"?

A. Deionized water 5%
B. Drug 5% in water
C. Dextrose 5% in water
D. Dispense 5% strength
E. Dilute to 5% strength

176. What is the meaning of the medical abbreviation "NS"

A. Natural solution
B. Nasal spray
C. Nasal solution
D. Normal saline
E. Normal strength

177. SIG or Signa is one of the basic parts of a prescription. Which of the following information is found in Signa?

A. Prescriber's information
B. Drug name and strength
C. Directions to be followed by the patient
D. Number of refills
E. Dispensing pharmacy information

178. A patient profile is an important record intended to enhance the safety of drug therapy. Which of the following information is NOT included in a patient's profile?

A. Date of birth
B. Social status
C. Gender
D. Known drug allergies
E. Full name

179. Which of the following drug related information is NOT included on a drug label?

A. Drug name
B. Drug strength
C. Quantity of drug dispensed
D. Drug-drug interactions
E. Drug expiration date

180. Acetone breath containing ketones is a characteristic of:

I. Type I diabetes
II. Type II diabetes
III. Diabetes insipidus

A. I only
B. III only
C. I and II only
D. II and III only
E. I, II, and III

181. Which of the following is a controlled drug part II?

A. Methadone
B. Phenobarbital
C. Tylenol #3
D. Amphetamine
E. Tylenol #4

182. All prescription for narcotics, narcotics preparations and other controlled drugs must be kept for at least:

A. 6 months
B. 12 months
C. 18 months
D. 24 months
E. 36 months

183. Correct statement concerning methylphenidate (Ritalin) prescription:

A. Refills are permitted for a verbal prescription if the prescriber has indicated the number of refills and dates
B. All refills require a new prescription
C. Refills are permitted for a written original prescription if the prescriber has indicated the number of refills and dates
D. Refills are permitted for verbal or written prescription if less than one year old
E. Refills are permitted for verbal or written prescription subject to professional discretion

Case study: Questions 184 to 185

PR is a 56-year-old woman with type 2 diabetes, hypertension, and dyslipidemia.
Her medications include metformin, glyburide, enteric-coated aspirin, lisinopril, HCTZ, and lovastatin. She developed an upper respiratory infection (URI) for which she was prescribed erythromycin, TID for 10 days.

184. What are possible drug-drug interactions?

A. Lovastatin-Lisinopril
B. Erythromycin-Lisinopril
C. Lovastatin-metformin
D. Erythromycin- Lovastatin
E. Lisinopril-Glyburide

185. Which of the following options would protect best this patient from a clinically significant drug interaction?

A. Stop taking lovastatin
B. Hold on lovastatin until the treatment of erythromycin is finished
C. Change her prescription to another antibiotic such as azithromycin
D. Change lovastatin prescription to atorvastatin
E. Change lovastatin prescriptilon to simvastatin

186. The auxiliary label of which of the following drugs may include "Empty stomach administration"?

    A. Sildenafil
    B. Carvedilol
    C. Risedronate
    D. Phenytoin
    E. Zolpidem

187. The auxiliary label of which of the following drugs may include "Do not crush tablet"?

    A. Methotrexate
    B. Ampicillin
    C. Captopril
    D. Sucralfate
    E. Zulepon

Case Study: Questions 188 to 190

Ms. John's profile is a 75-year-old Alzheimers's patient
Other conditions include Raynaud's phenomenon and hyperlipidemia
Allergies : Penicillin
Current Medications: Rivastigmine, nifedipine, ASA, lorazepam, pravastatin

188. Which of the following Alzheimer's drugs does not inhibit acetylcolinesterase?

   I. Memantine
  II. Rivastigmine
 III. Galantamine

    A. I only
    B. III only
    C. I and II only
    D. II and III only
    E. I, II, and III

189. Ms John's nutritionist reports that grapefruit juice is her regular beverage. Grapefruit juice should be avoided because it interacts with:

    A. ASA
    B. Donepezil
    C. Lorazepam
    D. Nifedipine
    E. Pravastatin

190. Which recommendation would be appropriate to best manage the grapefruit juice?

    A. Space apart the grapefruit juice and the interacting medication by at least 2 hours
    B. Discontinue the interacting medication since risks outweigh the benefits
    C. Switch to another medication to avoid side effects
    D. Monitor for increased levels and response of the interacting medication
    E. Discontinue the grapefruit juice

Answers

1. E

2. D
Raloxifene is an estrogen modulator that decreases the risk of breast cancer in high risk postmenopausal women. It is contraindicated in pregnant or lactating women, and in women with history of deep vein thrombosis. However, raloxifene has no effect of the levels of triglycerides and HDL.

3. D
Thrombocytopenia is one of the side effects of heparin.

4. E
Terazosin is a selective alpha 1 antagonist.

5. C
Coal tar is added to shampoo to treat dandruff and head lice.

6. C

7. D
Varenicline is nicotine receptor agonist whereas bupropion is antidepressant. Nicotine replacement formulations include gum, lozenges, patch, spray and inhaler.

8. C

9. D
Lindane is associated with neurotoxicity.

10. B
Hypertension is best treated with calcium channel blockers or diuretics in patients of African descent.

11. C

12. A

In case of penicillin resistance penicillinase-resistant beta lactam antibiotics such as oxacillin and flucloxacillin are preferred.

13. A

14. B

Cephalosporins in general should be used with cautious or avoided in patients with renal insufficiency. There is also high risk of aminoglycosides induced ototoxicity in patients with renal failure.

15. E

MRSA refer of S. aureus resistant to beta-lactam antibiotics. The remaining antibiotics are all used to treat MRSA infections however vancomycin is the drug of choice.

16. E

The use of quinolones is also associated with C. difficile infection.

17. A

18. C

Dyskinesia is another side effect of levodopa. Nystagmus is the side effect of phenytoin, carbamazepine and barbiturates.

19. B

Chloasma may be treated with hydroquinone.

20. C

21. C

Lovastatin can be taken BID.

22. A
Hydrochlorothiazide therapy leads to hypokalemia. Yellow vision is also called xanthopsia.

23. A
Atypical antipsychotics have lower incidence of extrapyramidal symptoms compared to typical antipsychotics.

24. E
Sulfapyridine has antibacterial effect whereas 5-ASA has anti-inflammatory effect.

25. E

26. B
Secondary dyslipidemia may be caused by several conditions including hypothyroidism, chronic renal failure, diabetes and pregnancy.

27. B
The following antibacterials are commonly associated with photosensitivity: quinolones, tetracyclines and sulfonamides

28. E
In general, statins are taken in the evening.

29. D
Dorzolamide is a carbonic anhydrase inhibitor that does not increase the toxicity of phenytoin. Phenytoin decreases the effectiveness of loop diuretics. Phenytoin is used to treat partial and generalized seizures, and status epilepticus if given by IV.

30. D
Phenytoin increases the metabolism of statins resulting in decreased lipid lowering effect. Pravastatin will be the safest for this patient since it is not metabolized by P450 enzymes.

31. A

32. B
The lack of effectiveness of ranitidine may be a sign of H. pylori infection.

33. D
Food products decrease the absorption of omeprazole by 35%.

34. C
The clearance of theophylline is also increased by phenytoin, phenobarbital and sulfinpyrazone.

35. B
Docusate is a stool softener with emulsifying and wetting properties. Avoid using docusate with mineral oil. Instead, use docusate with stimulant laxatives such as bisacodyl, cascara and senna. Avoid bulking agents including methylcellulose and psyllium in the treatment of opioid-induced constipation.

36. E
Store at 15C – 30C

37. B
Ethosuximide is used in the treatment of absence seizures.

38. B
In general, newer antidepressants such as bupropion, mirtazapine, nefazodone, trazodone and venlafaxine have less adverse effects.

39. D

40. D
Methotrexate may be added to any of the drugs listed above for enhanced effectiveness

41. C
Topiramate decreases body weight.

42. E
Coomb's test detects antibodies.

43. D
Stage I has almost no symptoms with the exception of occasional vomiting; nausea, vomiting and abdominal pain are likely in stage II; stage III is characterized by bleeding and malfunction of liver, kidneys and pancreas.

44. E
Senna and phenazopyridine discolor urine as well.

45. B
Phenytoin is also linked to increased liver enzymes, blood dyscrasias (blood disorders) and coarse facial appearance with long-term use.

46. E

47. A

48. E

49. D
Clavulanate inhibits beta lactamase resulting in decreased degradation of amoxicillin.

50. C

51. A
Chlorthalidone and furosemide are diuretics and cause metabolic alkalosis. Miglitol is antihyperglycemic.

52. E

53. E
They increase urine glucose level resulting in false positive response.
Chloramphenicol has the same effect.

54. A
Potassium iodide is also used to treat hyperthyroidism. Its absorption is
decreased by dairy products.

55. C

56. C
Grapefruit juice may increase the adverse effects of nifedipine.

57. E
One of the common adverse effects of ACE inhibitors used as antihypertensives
is dry cough.

58. C
The dose has to be loaded prior to administration. Always check the dose
counter.

59. E
Dry mouth, nose and eyes are common side effects. Accutane (isotretinoin)
increases blood lipids as well.

60. C
Flucytosine is antifungal

61. E

62. C
Calcium and vitamin D supplements are recommended during raloxifene therapy.

63. D

64. D

Other risk factors are menopause and lack of exercise. Obesity is a risk factor for arthritis.

65. D

66. D

Iron deficiency is the leading cause of anemia.

67. E

Conjuctivitis can be also caused by viruses, allergies and irritants such as chemicals. Other antibacterials used are: gentamicin, tobramycin, ciprofloxacin, erythromycin, neomycin, ofloxacin, trimethoprim and polymycin B combo.

68. C

Voltaren contains diclofenac and is used to decrease pain, swelling and inflammation.

69. B

70. C

Other non-benzodiazepine hypnotics include zolpidem, zaleplon and indiplon.

71. E

Other side effects of methotrexate include blurred vision, headache, thrombocytopenia, photosensitivity, alopecia, depigmentation or hyperpigmentation, ulcerative stomatitis and osteoporosis. Methotrexate is indicated for the treatment of cancer, rheumatoid arthritis and severe psoriasis resistant to other treatments.

72. D

HRT is also contraindicated in patients with hormone dependent cancer.

73. E

HRT can also help relieve anxiety and depression.

74. D

75. E

76. A
Iron is best absorption on empty stomach when acidity is the highest.

77. C
Vertical flow hood is best suited for handling carcinogenic products.

78. A

79. C
Lugol's solution is made by dissolving 5g of iodine and 10 g of potassium iodide in distilled water up to a total volume of 100 mL. Tincture of iodine which is another disinfectant contains a mix of water and alcohol. Chiller's test is used in the diagnosis of cervical cancer. Lugol's solution is also used in the treatment of hyperthyroidism; take with food or milk to reduce GI irritation.

80. B

81. C
A second dose may be given is symptoms persist but at least 2 hours after the first dose.

82. B

83. B

84. A
Killed vaccines including cholera, rabies and hepatitis A do not require refrigeration.

85. E

86. C
Anthracycline chemotherapeutics including daunorubicin and epirubucin are associated with cardiotoxicity.

87. E
The most common side effects are bone pain and fever.

88. E

89. E
Infliximab is a therapeutic monoclonal antibody. DMARD stands for disease-modifying antirrheumatic drug.

90. D

91. B

92. D
Infliximab and adalimumab are used to treat autoimmune disorders; Muromonab is used to prevent transplant rejection; Abciximab is used to treat cardiovascular conditions.

93. C
It becomes effective 10 days after the injection for duration of three years.

94. C

95. C

96. E

97. D
EDTA is an example of chelating agent.

98. E
The process is called forced alkaline diuresis.

99. B

100. C

101. C
Milliequivalent weight (mEq.wt) = Molecular weight of an atom or radical (ion) in g / valence (or charge) of the atom or radical x 1000
The molecular weight of sodium is 58.44 and it has a valence of 1
Therefore 3 mEq = 3 x 58.44 / 1 x 1000 = 0.175 g
Since we have 0.175 g in 1 mL the strength of the solution is 17.5%

102. B
Step 1: calculate the amount of drug needed per min
5 ug x 75 kg = 375 ug /min
Step 2: calculate the volume per min using the concentration provided
V = 375 / 400 = 0.93 mL/min

103. A
Midazolam and triazolam are short acting; Alprazolam, clonazepam, lorazepam, oxazepam and temazepam are intermediate acting; Diazepam, flurazepam and chlordiazepoxide are long acting.

104. D
Midazolam is another useful treatment for status epilepticus.

105. B
Petit mal also called absence seizures is characterized by loss of awareness.

106. E
Sulfinpyrazone, probenecid and allopurinol are uricosuric drugs; they decrease blood levels of uric acid. They are used for prevention NOT in acute attack.

107. B
ACE inhibitors and alpha blockers are preferred for diabetic patients. Same for patients with heart failure.

108. B

109. D

110. B

111. A
Low molecular weight heparins are used as well.

112. D
Nevirapine, efavirenz and delavirdine are non-nucleoside reverse transcriptase inhibitors.

113. E
Carpal tunnel syndrome results from the thickening and damage of connective tissues. Kidney failure and nephropathy are other complications of diabetes.

114. E
Narrow therapeutic index means that the amount of drug needed to provide therapeutic benefit is close to the amount of drug that leads to toxicity. Therapeutic drug monitoring is required.

115. A

116. C
Bimatoprost is s prostaglandin-like compound given as eye drop.

117. B
Cholinergic drugs are used instead because anticholinergic drugs cause mydriasis (pupil dilation).

118. E
Dyskinea seen in Parkinson's patients results from chronic levodopa (L-dopa) therapy.

119. D
Carbidopa inhibits peripheral conversion of levodopa to dopamine due to the inhibition of DOPA carboxylase.

120. E

121. B
Long term hydrocortisone therapy leads to hyperglycemia by antagonizing the effect of insulin. Electrolyte unbalance leading to fluid retention and edema is another adverse effect of long term hydrocortisone therapy.

122. F
A keratolytic agent causes the outer layer of skin to loosen and shed resulting in improved moisture.

123. C
Bone thinning is caused by vitamin D deficiency; sore tongue is caused by vitamin B2 deficiency; bleeding gums is caused by vitamin C deficiency; tendency to bleed is caused by vitamin K deficiency.

124. E
Diuretics decrease fluid retention resulting in decreased edema.

125. D

126. C
Verapamil and diltiazem are nondihydropyridine CCBs whereas nifidipine, nicardipine and amlodipine are dihydropyridine CCBs.

127. D

Hemochromatosis is characterized by high transferrin saturation and serum ferritin levels.

128. C
Ivermectin is used for the treatment of roundworm infection.

129. B
Tissue necrosis is also due to cancer, injury and poisons. Apoptosis is a naturally occurring cell death.

130. E
Prostaglandins, leukotrienes and histamine are pro-inflammatory, antipyretics decrease fever whereas pyrogens are fever inducers.

131. D
The onset of acute inflammation is immediate but delayed in chronic inflammation.
Inflammation is characterized by redness, pain, swelling, heat and loss of function.

132. D
Cholecystitis is often caused by the presence of gallstones in the gallbladder which results in blockage of the cystic duct.

133. C
The metabolism of a prodrug produces an active metabolite. Acyclovir, levodopa, heroin, codeine, enalapril, fosphenytoin and prednisone are also prodrugs.

134. A
Pyrantel pamoate and ivermectin are primarily effective against nematodes; albendazole and mebendazole are effective against both nematodes and cestodes; praziquantel is effective against trematodes and cestodes;

135. D
Tinea pedis is also called athlete's foot.

136. C
The combo atovaquone/proguanil is the most effective and treatment should start only 1 day prior to visiting a malaria-endemic area and 7 days afterwards.

137. E
Pectin is another adsorbent. The remaining agents are intestinal muscle relaxants used to treat diarrhea.

138. C
Common side effects include abdominal cramps, diarrhea and nausea.

139. D
Sorbitol is an osmotic agent used also to treat constipation.

140. B
The clearance of theophilline is also decreased by propranolol, allopurinol and erythromycin.

141. A

142. E

143. A

144. C

145. B
Epinephrine is also use when an acute asthma attack is not responsive to salbutamol. Diphenhydramine is used to treat severe allergic reactions.

146. C
Ipratopium is anticholinergic used usually in combination with beta agonists.

147. B
This class of asthma drugs includes beclomethasone, budesonide, fluticasone and triamcinolone. They are effective in the prevention (long term control) of asthma.

148. C
This class of antibiotics includes amikacin, gentamicin, kanamycin and streptomycin.

149. E
Ceftazidime is a third generation cephalosporin; nafcillin is a penicillin; sulfacetamide is a sulfonamide.

150. E

151. C
A → Tylenol #1; B → Tylenol #3; D → Tylenol #4

152. B
The process is called forced acid diuresis. Forced acid diuresis is effective because amphetamine is basic. Hyperthermia and hyperactivity are signs of amphetamine overdose.

153. D

154. B
p.m. means evening or afternoon

155. E

156. A

157. C
St. John's wort decreases digoxin bioavailability resulting in decreased effectiveness.

158. A
Theophylline leads to activation of peptic ulcer; cigarette smoking decreases the clearance the theophylline resulting in increased effectiveness.

159. D
Therapeutic choice is another useful reference.

160. B
Steatorrhea is oily and loose stools. Orlistat lacks effectiveness if the patient has a diet with less than 30% fat.

161. C
Orlistat is taken during a meal or up to one hour following a meal.

162. E

163. C
Licorice increases the loss of potassium. Saw Palmetto increases the effectiveness of hormone replacement therapy (HRT) and oral contraceptives.

164. A
SPF stands for Sun Protection Factor.

165. E
It is recommended to start with full strength patch then decrease gradually.

166. B
Rifampin is used to treat tuberculosis and leprosy (Hansen's disease). Conjunctivitis, heartburn, and soreness of mouth and tongue are other adverse effects of rifampin.

167. C
Biopharmaceuticals include proteins and nucleic acid drugs. They are also called biologics or biotherapeutics or biotechnology drugs.

168. B
When solving percentage problems use the following formula

IF # parts / 100 = THEN Amount of solute needed / Total volume or weight of product

169. D
When solving dilution problems use the following formula

D1 x C1 = D2 x C2

D1 = volume or weight of stock solution
C1 = concentration of stock solution
D2 = volume or weight of desired solution
C2 = concentration of desired solution

Note: D1 and D2 must be in the same units; C1 and C2 must be in the same units

170. A
Alligation problem.
To solve this problem, follow the steps below.

1. Draw a problem matrix

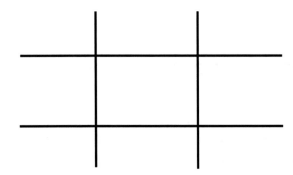

2. Insert quantities as shown

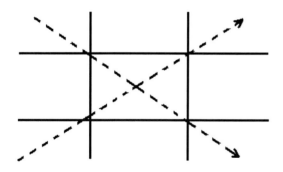

Highest strength

Desired strength

Lowest strength

3. Subtract along the diagonals

4. Read along the horizontals

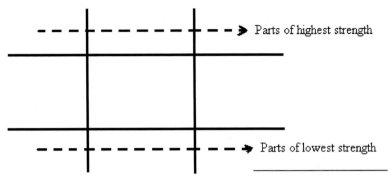

Parts of highest strength

Parts of lowest strength

The sum equals the number
of parts of desired strength

171. B

172. D

173. C

174. E

175. C

176. D

177. C

178. B

179. D

180. A

181. B

182. D

183. C

184. D
Erythromycin increases blood level of statins due to the inhibition of CYP3A4.

185. C
Azithromycin does not interact with statins. Among statins, pravastastin has low potential of drug interaction since it is not metabolized by P450 enzymes. Fluvastatin and rosuvastatin have less interaction with erythromycin since they are primarily metabolized by CYP2C9 not CYP3A4.

186. C

187. A

188. A
Memantine is N-methyl-D-aspartate (NMDA) receptor antagonist.

189. D

190. E

BEHAVIOURAL SOCIAL AND ADMINISTRATIVE PHARMACY SCIENCES

Questions

1. NAPRA stands for:

A. National Association of Pharmacy Representatives Administration
B. National Association of Pharmacy Regulatory Authorities
C. National Association of Provincial Regulatory Authorities
D. National Association of Provincial Representatives Administration
E. National Association of Pharmacy Regulatory Agencies

2. Verbal communication is essential in a pharmacy setting. Which of the following attributes of verbal communication is the MOST important?

A. Accuracy of the message
B. Tone of voice
C. Voice pitch
D. Choice of words
E. Face-to-face

3. According to PIPEDA, which of the following are considered confidential information?

I. Opinions
II. Social status
III. Income

A. I only
B. III only
C. I and II only
D. II and III only
E. I, II, and III

4. Nonverbal communication is a very important method of sending messages. This form of communication is underestimated in many cases. Which of the following is NOT a feature of nonverbal communication?

    A. Personal space
    B. Smiling
    C. Facial expressions
    D. Choice of words
    E. Eye contact

5. In healthcare which of the following costs is intangible?

    A. Cost of training staff
    B. Cost of needles
    C. Cost of equipment
    D. Cost of anxiety
    E. Cost of compounding

6. Which of the following financial statements describes the pharmacy assets, liabilities and owner's equity at a given point in time?

    A. Balance sheet
    B. Income statement
    C. Retained earnings
    D. Cash flow
    E. Profit and loss statement

7. Which of the following financial statements describes the pharmacy sales over a period of time?

    A. Balance sheet
    B. Income statement
    C. Retained earnings
    D. Cash flow
    E. Profit and loss statement

8. Which of the following financial terms measures the ability of a pharmacy to pay its liabilities at due time?

    A. Sales
    B. Equity
    C. Liquidity
    D. Inventory
    E. Account receivables

9. Which of the following substances is NOT regulated as precursor for illicit drug under the Precursor Control Regulations of the Controlled Drugs and Substances Act?

    A. Ergotamine
    B. Ephedra
    C. Lorazepam
    D. Norephedrine
    E. Ergometrine

10. The ethical principle of justice requires that the pharmacist:

    A. Respect the patient's right to make decisions
    B. Act with honesty without deception
    C. Prevent or remove harm
    D. Do good to patients
    E. Act with fairness and equality

11. Which of the following statements refers to the ethical principle of non-maleficence?

    A. Respect the patient's right to make decisions
    B. Act with honesty without deception
    C. Prevent or remove harm
    D. Do good to patients
    E. Act with fairness and equality

12. Recently, two pharmacy technicians have been dealing with strong disagreement. Which of the following is NOT an appropriate strategy to help solve the problem?

    A. Pharmacy manager assistance
    B. Avoidance of communication
    C. Management of emotions
    D. Transform the problem into learning opportunity
    E. Address the problem not individuals involved

13. For which of the following drugs the pharmacist will require a written prescription?

    A. Tylenol #4
    B. Tylenol #2
    C. Diazepam
    D. Butorphanol
    E. Testosterone

14. Correct statement regarding the ethical principle of justice:

    A. Act with fairness and equality
    B. Act with honesty
    C. Do good to patients
    D. Prevent or remove harm
    E. Respect patient's right to make decisions

15. Who is primarily responsible for drug procurement and inventory management in a pharmacy?

    A. Pharmacy technician
    B. Pharmacy intern
    C. Any pharmacist
    D. Pharmacy assistant
    E. Pharmacy manager

16. All of the following are required on a drug label, EXCEPT:

A. Name of the prescriber
B. Name of the patient
C. Refills schedule
D. The date the prescription is dispensed
E. Drug strength

17. A pharmacy has recently experienced a noticeable decrease in sales. What will be the best way to reduce the pharmacy expenses?

   A. Ordering less expensive drugs
   B. Reduce the number of pharmacy technicians
   C. Reduce staff hourly wage
   D. Reduce pharmacists overlap
   E. Reduce pharmacists work hours

18. When dealing with a drug dispensing error, which of the following is the least concern of the pharmacy manager?

   A. Discuss the situation with the staff involved
   B. Assess the situation
   C. Increase the frequency of staff training
   D. Consider the integration of automation in dispensing
   E. Notify Health Canada

19. Based on the following medications data which of the following antibiotics would be the most appropriate choice for a hospital pharmacy?

Antibiotic	Cost per day	Dosing Frequency	Length of treatment in days
I	$2.25	BID	7
II	$2.35	Once daily	14
III	$5.00	BID	10
IV	$2.50	BID	7
V	$ 3.75	Once daily	15

228

A. Antibiotic I
B. Antibiotic II
C. Antibiotic III
D. Antibiotic IV
E. Antibiotic V

20. A pharmacy turnover rate is a measure of:

A. Efficacy
B. Profit
C. Equity
D. Liquidity
E. Assets

21. DIN stand for:

A. Drug identification number
B. Dispensing index number
C. Drug identification name
D. Dispensing identification number
E. Drug index name

22. A management style is the overall method of leadership used by the manager. The style of management in which the pharmacy manager designs detailed policies and written procedures for employees to follow is called:

A. Consultative
B. Autocratic.
C. Bureaucratic.
D. Benevolent
E. Dictatorial

23. Which of the following describes the role of NAPRA:

A. Implementation of pharmacy practice standards across Canada
B. Promotion of universal health care in Canada
C. Regulation of the financial performance of provincial regulatory authorities
D. Protection of the rights of pharmacists
E. Promotion of the mandate of Health Canada

24. POS stands for:

A. Point of sale
B. Point of submission
C. Point of selection
D. Product on sale
E. Point of source

25. A 35 years old female with a chronic condition is refusing an experimental treatment which may prolonged her life. Her husband insists that the health care provider gives her the experimental drug. Which of the following ethical principle gives the health care provider the right NOT to provide the treatment?

A. Confidentiality
B. Veracity
C. Autonomy
D. Justice
E. Beneficence

26. All of the following are known as the 4Ps of marketing system, EXCEPT:

A. Price
B. Place
C. Product
D. Personnel
E. Promotion

27. Correct statements regarding pharmaceutical care:

I. Pharmaceutical care is a process of drug therapy management involving the pharmacist and patient's physician
II. The principles of pharmaceutical care are embedded in the concept of Good Pharmacy Practice
III. The goal of Pharmaceutical Care is to optimize the patient's health-related quality of life and achieve positive clinical outcomes within realistic economic expenditures

A. I only
B. III only
C. I and II only
D. II and III only
E. I, II, and III

28. The ethical principle of veracity requires that the pharmacist:

A. Respect the patient's right to make decisions
B. Act with honesty without deception
C. Do good to patients
D. Act with fairness
E. Prevent or remove harm

29. The ethical principle of autonomy requires that the pharmacist:

A. Respect the patient's right to make decisions
B. Act with honesty without deception
C. Prevent or remove harm
D. Act with fairness
E. Prevent or remove harm

30. Which of the following financial statements provides information on changes of pharmacy assets, liquidity, equity and liabilities over a period of time?

A. Income statement
B. Balance sheet
C. Cash flow
D. Return on investment
E. Gross income

31. BA is a regular patient who pays a fixed monthly amount for her health insurance. This amount is called:

A. Repayment
B. Balance
C. Copayment
D. Claim
E. Deductible

32. The clinical study of an antibiotic used as standard in the treatment of Otitis Media results in 94% cure rate in one week. A new antibiotic results in 97% cure rate in one week. What is relative risk reduction with the new drug?

A. 0.30
B. 0.69
C. 0.98
D. 1.03
E. 1. 75

$$\frac{0.97}{0.94} = \frac{3}{97} = \frac{3}{100}$$

33. Which of the following is the primary attribute of effective communication skills?

    A. Pitch of voice
    B. Personal space
    C. Tone of voice
    D. Choice of words
    E. Listening

34. All of the following statements are correct regarding adulterated drugs, EXCEPT:

    I. Prepared under unsanitary conditions not conformed to GMPs
    II. OTC drugs not packaged in tamper-resistant container
    III. Have a misleading label

    A. I only
    B. III only
    C. I and II only
    D. II and III only
    E. I, II, and III

35. Drug monographs also called package inserts provide detailed drug information. Which of the following is NOT listed in a drug monograph?

    A. Adverse effects
    B. Organic synthesis
    C. Dosage
    D. Chemical structure
    E. Pharmacokinetic studies

36. JN is moving permanently from British Columbia to Alberta. JN will be able to transfer his health insurance to Alberta based on which of Canada Health Act (CHA) principles?

A. Universality
B. Accessibility
C. Comprehensiveness
D. Public administration
E. Portability

37. The assessment of two drug therapeutic regimens with different success rates in achieving the same clinical outcome follows:

A. Cost effectiveness analysis (CEA)
B. Cost utility analysis (CUA)
C. Cost minimization analysis (CMA)
D. Cost benefit analysis (CBA)

Case Study: Questions 38 to 39

Mrs. John is visiting the pharmacy to get her last refill for atorvastatin. She receives her medication from a pharmacy technician who failed to remind her that she has no refills left.

38. Which of the following principles has been violated?

    A. Veracity
    B. Confidentiality
    C. Beneficience
    D. Autonomy
    E. Justice

39. 4 weeks later, Mrs John returned to the pharmacy for a refill. The pharmacist realized that she has no refill left. Which of the following will be an appropriate action?

    A. Refuse to provide a refill and ask her to get a new prescription
    B. Refills are not permitted for atorvastatin
    C. Provide a refill and call her physician to renew her prescription
    D. Provide a refill and ask her to return to the pharmacy with a new prescription within 48 hours
    E. Call her physician then wait until the prescription is faxed before providing a refill

40. Which of the following is NOT a responsibility of the pharmacy technician?

    A. Perform final check prior to releasing a drug
    B. Receive a prescription
    C. Prepare medication for release
    D. Transfer a prescription
    E. Perform pharmaceutical calculations

41. Which of the following is NOT included in the duties of a pharmacy technician?

    A. Call an insurance company on behalf of a patient
    B. Accept a refill order
    C. Provide advice on drug adverse effects
    D. Request a refill order
    E. Check a drug formulation prepared by another pharmacy technician

42. Which of the following clinical trials phases is post-marketing?

A. Phase 1
B. Phase 2
C. Phase 3
D. Phase 4

43. The ethical principle of beneficence required that pharmacists:

A. Do good to the patient
B. Remove or prevent harm to the patient
C. Respect the patient's right to make choices
D. Act with fairness
E. Be honest

44. Correct statements regarding the statistical error type II:

I. Data shows no difference between two experimental treatments but there is actually a difference *β eror = false negative type II*
II. Data shows a difference between two experimental treatments but there is actually no difference *(type I) = false positive (α eror)*
III. p (probability) value < 0.05 is the level of significance

P > 0.05 = level of significance

A. I only
B. III only
C. I and II only
D. II and III only
E. I, II, and III

45. An investigational drug clinical trial results showed that the symptoms of patients taking the drug have improved compared to patients taking a placebo with a p value of -0.9. What best describes these results?

A. The drug is more effective than the placebo
B. The drug is less effective than the placebo
C. There is no difference between the drug and the placebo
D. There is high incidence of type I error
E. There is high incidence of alpha error

46. The principle of universal access to health care in Canada is the mandate of:

A. Canada Research based Pharmaceutical Companies
B. Provincial and Territorial Pharmacy Regulatory Authorities
C. Provincial and Territorial Health Authorities
D. Canada Health Act
E. National Association of Pharmacy Regulatory Authorities

47. Which of the following is NOT a principle of Canadian Health Act?

    A. Portability
    B. Universality
    C. Comprehensiveness
    D. Accessibility
    E. Private administration

48. The loss or theft of targeted substances must be reported primarily to:

    A. Provincial or Territorial Pharmacy Regulatory Authority (copy)
    B. Federal Minister of Health
    C. Drug Manufacturer
    D. Local Police
    E. Local pharmacies

49. According to the Personal Information Protection and Electronic Documents Act (PIPEDA), which of the following statement is NOT correct?

    A. The purpose of collecting the information must be identified
    B. Collected information must be stored in a secured place
    C. If requested, the patient must have access to her information
    D. Collected information must not be disclosed without patient's consent even when required by law

50. SAP stands for:

    A. Special approval program
    B. Special access program
    C. Special approval policy
    D. Special access policy

51. Which of the following organization ensures that the cost of patented drugs is not excessive in Canada?

    A. CGPA
    B. ISMP
    C. PMPRB
    D. NDMAC
    E. NAPRA

52. The destruction of targeted drugs must be witnessed and records must be kept for at least:

    A. 6 months
    B. 1 year
    C. 18 months
    D. 2 years
    E. 3 years

53. The loss of theft of targeted substances must be reported to the Federal Minister of Health within:

    A. 10 days
    B. 2 weeks
    C. 1 month
    D. 2 months
    E. 3 months

54. Total sales of a pharmacy in 2008 are estimated at $850,000. The overall expenses for the same year are $585,000. What is the pharmacy gross profit?

A. $425,000
B. $ 350,000
C. $ 265,000
D. $85,000

55. Correct statements regarding Schedule I drugs:

I. Require a prescription for sale and are provided to the public by the pharmacist
II. Sale is controlled in a regulated environment as defined by provincial pharmacy legislation.
III. Include vaccines, insulin and oxymetazoline nasal spray

    A. I only
    B. III only
    C. I and II only
    D. II and III only
    E. I, II, and III

56. Which of the following formula represents a pharmacy net income?

A. Gross income + fixed assets
B. Total sales - liquidity
C. Gross income – expenses including taxes
D. Total sales + current assets
E. Gross income – staff salary

57. All of the following are found in the Food and Drugs Act schedule D, EXCEPT:

    A. Vaccines
    B. Insulin
    C. Antibodies
    D. Blood derivatives
    E. Radiopharmaceuticals

Case Study: Questions 58-59

TG who is dating your best friend comes to your pharmacy with a prescription for HIV drugs. You begin to worry that your friend isn't aware of his condition.

58. Which of the following would be an appropriate step?

    A. Arrange a meeting with both TG and your friend to discuss his condition
    B. Urge TG to inform your friend about his diagnosis
    C. Disclose to your friend that TG is being treated for HIV
    D. Refrain from telling your friend about his condition but advise her to always use safe sex measures and to be checked for HIV if she has had unprotected sex
    E. You trust that TG is responsible enough to tell you friend

59. Which of the following statements guides you BEST in resolving this dilemma?

    A. A pharmacist is obliged to protect the patient's right of confidentiality, if the patient is capable of making rational decisions
    B. A pharmacist may breach confidentiality when failure to disclose information will place other persons in serious danger
    C. The burden is on TG. He will probably act accordingly
    D. TG's physician should ensure the patient understands the importance of preventing the spread of the disease
    E. You have to protect the welfare of your best friend

60. Which of the following statement characterizes empty stomach administration?

    A. Anytime before a meal
    B. 15 minutes before a meal
    C. 30 minutes before a meal
    D. 45 minutes before a meal
    E. 1 hours before a meal

61. A pharmacist is making a presentation on the risks of improper disposal of drugs. He may discuss the following strategies, EXCEPT:

A. Implementation of drug disposable process involving other community pharmacies
B. Documentation of the amount of expired drugs collected
C. Documentation of the amount of unused not expired drugs collected
D. Encouraging patients to return unused and expired drugs to the manufacturer
E. Promotion of community involvement

62. All of the following are included in a pharmacy total assets, EXCEPT:

A. Value of building
B. Total value of equipment
C. Expenses including taxes
D. Account receivables
E. Inventory

63. All of the following are types of pharmacy ownership, EXCEPT:

I.   Franchise
II. Incorporation
III. Leasing

A. I only
B. III only
C. I and II only
D. II and III only
E. I, II, and III

64. A cancer patient was concerned about losing her hair during the course of the treatment. The pharmacist confirmed her fears and explained that it is a common side effect due to the toxicity of cancer drugs. Which of the following principles has been followed?

A. Justice
B. Autonomy
C. Beneficience
D. Veracity
E. Non-maleficence

65. A patient asks his pharmacist for assistance regarding the proper use of an inhaler. Instead of providing counseling, the pharmacist advised the patient to follow the instructions provided. Which of the following principles has been violated?

    A. Non-maleficience
    B. Beneficience
    C. Veracity
    D. Justice
    E. Autonomy

66. Which of the following statements are correct regarding standard deviation?

    I. Used to evaluate the accuracy of data
    II. Measures the dispersion of data point from the mean
    III. Equals the square root of the variance

        A. I only
        B. III only
        C. I and II only
        D. II and III only
        E. I, II, and III

67. Which of the following statements describes best the "Student's test"?

    A. Continuous probability distribution that describes data that clusters around the mean
    B. Statistical significance of the difference between two means
    C. Parametric test use to evaluate the true value of a parameter based on a sample
    D. Non-parametric test for assessing whether two independent observations come from the same distribution
    E. Compares statistical models in order to identify the model that best fits the population being investigated

Answers

1. B
NAPRA is an association of provincial and territorial pharmacy regulatory bodies as well as the Canadian Forces Pharmacy Services. NAPRA facilitates the adoption and implementation of regulatory practices across Canada.

2. A

3. E

4. D
Other features of nonverbal communication include posture, gestures and silence.

5. D
Costs of needles and compounding are direct costs; costs of training staff and equipment are indirect costs.

6. A

7. B

8. C

9. C
Other controlled precursors under the act are: ephedrine and pseudoephedrine.

10. E

11. C

12. B

13. A

Written OR verbal prescription for tylenol #2, diazepam, butorphanol and testosterone.

14. A

15. E

16. C

17. D

18. E

19. A

The decision is based on drug efficacy and cost.

20. A

The turnover rate is a measure of how quickly the inventory is sold.

21. A

The DIN is assigned by Health Canada

22. C

Autocratic refers to implementing owns opinions without any consultation. In consultative management style the pharmacy staff provides views and opinions.

23. A

24. A

25. C

26. D

27. E

28. B

29. A

30. C

31. C

32. D
The relative risk is the risk of an event relative to exposure = 0.97/0.94

33. E

34. B
Drugs with false or misleading label are called misbranded. Drugs packaged in non-sterile or contaminated containers are also adulterated.

35. B
Additional information found in a typical drug monograph includes clinical pharmacology, indications, contraindications, warnings, precautions, abuse and dependence potential, and formulation.

36. E
All five are principles of Canada Health Act (CHA).

37. A

38. C

39. C
Because atorvastatin belongs to schedule F.

40. A
Final check prior to release must be performed by a pharmacist

41. C

42. D
Phases 1, 2 and 3 are performed pre-marketing to test the safety of the drug and to indentify the required therapeutic dosage. Phase 4 refers to long term assessment of drug safety following approval.

43. A

44. A
II refers to statistical error type I or false positive or alpha error. Type II error or false negative or beta error; p value equal or lower than 0.05 means that type I error is unlikely. p value > 0.05 is the level of significance.

45. A

46. D

47. E
Public administration not private administration.

48. B
A copy of the report must be forwarded to provincial or territorial pharmacy regulatory authority.

49. D

50. B
SAP provides access to not yet approved drugs and is managed by Health Canada.

51. C
CGPA: Canadian Generic Pharmaceutical Association; ISMP: Institute of Safe Medication Practices; PMPRB: Patented Medicines Prices Review Board; NDMAC: Non-prescription Drug Manufacturers Association of Canada.

52. D

53. A

54. C
Gross Profit = Sales – Expenses (excluding taxes)
Net Profit = Gross Profit – Taxes = Gross Profit – Total Expenses (including taxes)

55. C
Vaccine and insulin are schedule II drugs and oxymetazoline nasal spray is unscheduled.

56. C

57. E
Radiopharmaceuticals are found in schedule C.

58. D

59. A

60. E
Empty stomach administration requires drug administration 1 hour before **OR** 2 hours after a meal

61. D

62. C

63. C
Sole proprietorship is another form of ownership.

64. D

65. B

66. E

67. B
A refers to normal distribution or Gaussian distribution; C refers to Wald test; D refers to Wilcoxon-Mann-Whitney test; E refers to F-test.

CPSIA information can be obtained at www.ICGtesting.com
Printed in the USA
LVOW031659200512

282475LV00001BA/6/P